Reclaiming Sex & Intimacy After Prostate Cancer

A Guide for Men and Their Partners

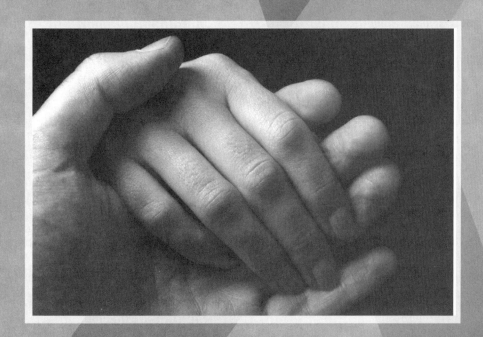

Jeffrey Albaugh, PhD, APRN, CUCNS

ISBN: 978-0-9846597-1-5

Publication Management by
Anthony J. Jannetti, Inc., East Holly Avenue, Box 56, Pitman, NJ 08071-0056
856-256-2300; FAX 856-589-7463; www.ajj.com

DISCLAIMER

The author and publisher of this book have made serious efforts to ensure that treatments, practices, and procedures are accurate and conform to standards accepted at the time of publication. Due to constant changes in information resulting from continuing research and clinical experience, reasonable differences in opinions among authorities, unique aspects of individual clinical situations, and the possibility of human error in preparing such a publication require that the reader exercise individual judgment when making a clinical decision, and if necessary, consult and compare information from other authorities, professionals, or sources.

Table of Contents

Chapter

Acknowledgment

This book was made possible by the very generous financial support of William D. and Pamela Hutul Ross and John and Carol Walter through funding from the NorthShore University Healthcare System Foundation. It is individuals such as these who make it possible to disseminate important educational information to empower men with prostate cancer and their partners to make informed and educated choices. I cannot thank them enough for sharing my vision for creating this book, which would not have been published without their crucial support.

I am so thankful to many other people who also helped me with the book. Several people helped review the manuscript and gave me input at various points in the process. I would like to thank experts Martha McCurdy, Dr. Peter Colegrove, Dr. Charles B. Brendler, Jean Lewis, Dr. Linda Sizemore, Dulce Bramblett, and the prostate cancer survivors for their help in reviewing and providing input. Thank you to Robert and Keely Hillison for reviewing my contract. I would like to thank the entire staff of Anthony J. Jannetti, Inc., including my Editor Ken Thomas. I would truly like to thank my wife Julie for putting up with the many hours I have spent on the road educating patients and health care professionals and writing this book about sex after prostate cancer. I could not have done it without her support and love; she is simply the best. I want to thank my sons Nathan and Kyle for helping out at home when I am on the road or busy with work. I have been blessed with so many people in my life who have encouraged and supported me throughout my career including Joe and Carol Albaugh (my parents), my sisters Jo and Lisa, my best friend since grade school Gina Keeven, my dear friends Tracy and Tom Ceseretti, and the many other friends and family (you all know who you are and I love each of you) who have encouraged me. Most of all I would like to thank God for giving my life purpose and meaning through my work with the incredible patients who I am honored to help in their journey towards maximal quality of life.

Dedication

This book is dedicated to the amazing patients I have cared for and their partners who have taught me so much about courageously fighting to improve quality of life after prostate cancer.

Foreword

When I first met Jeff Albaugh several years ago, I was impressed not only by his expertise in sexual health, but, even more so, by his remarkable energy and enthusiasm for his chosen profession. I, therefore, made it a priority to recruit Dr. Albaugh to NorthShore University HealthSystem (NorthShore) so that we could work together to build a sexual health program. Dr. Albaugh and I share the same caring approach to patients that creates a different kind of nurturing environment focused on maximizing quality of life for patients and their partners. Since I met Jeff, he has not only built a successful clinical practice, but he has also established strong collaborative relationships with our colleagues in other medical disciplines including gynecology, family practice, internal medicine, and physical therapy. Earlier this year, through the generosity of Mr. and Mrs. William Ross, the NorthShore Ross Clinic for Sexual Health was established. This clinic is unique in the Chicagoland area and is one of only a few facilities in the United States that provides comprehensive care for both men and women with sexual health concerns.

It is indeed a pleasure to write the Foreward for Jeff's book, which is long overdue. *All* treatments for prostate cancer can result in diminished sexual health. Prior to treatment, physicians understandably emphasize the importance of cancer cure, while minimizing the significant sexual effects that are associated with prostate cancer treatments. Similarly, patients are understandably frightened by the diagnosis of prostate cancer and are either unaware or reluctant to discuss this issue before undergoing treatment. Following treatment, however, when the fear of cancer is diminished, this very important quality-of-life issue assumes much greater significance, and, unfortunately, physicians again may minimize sexual health concerns, and, at best, address these issues reluctantly and superficially.

This book should be read by all men, as well as their partners, prior to undergoing prostate cancer treatment. In a clear and patient-friendly style supplemented with numerous illustrative diagrams and sidebar highlights to emphasize important "take home messages," Dr. Albaugh discusses the risks to sexual health associated with each type of treatment for prostate cancer, and then addresses the specific risks associated with surgery, including dry orgasms and shrinkage of the penis. He then provides a thorough overview of all available treatments for erectile dysfunction, devotes separate chapters to each of these treatments, and also provides a discussion regarding the post-treatment strategy of penile rehabilitation. The book concludes with two chapters devoted to the importance of psychological well-being to normal sexual function and a very supportive chapter for the partners of men dealing with sexual dysfunction following prostate cancer treatment.

I am indeed both proud and fortunate to work with Dr. Albaugh, and I know that this book will be an invaluable resource for all men with prostate cancer and their partners.

Charles B. Brendler, MD
Co-Director, John and Carol Walter Center for Urological Health & William and
*   Pamela Hutul Ross Clinic for Sexual Health*
NorthShore University HealthSystem
Evanston, IL

Chapter 1
Introduction

Sometimes the road towards healing can be a challenging journey. You probably never thought you would be reading this book. You may be overwhelmed from your prostate cancer diagnosis. You may fear you will never have sex again. You may feel guilty for worrying about sex after your prostate cancer diagnosis. Yet, the things you are feeling are very normal and there is hope. You *can* continue to have a fulfilling relationship with your partner. You *can* reclaim intimacy and closeness with your partner. This book is dedicated to you and your partner or future partner. So where and how do you begin this journey of reclamation? You begin by increasing your knowledge about sex and intimacy.

Sex, Intimacy, and Communication

There are many definitions of sex and several things may come to mind when you think about sex. Sex is often thought of as the act of sex or those characteristics of being male or female. Sex is typically thought of in terms of genitals and arousing stimulation. Genital stimulation can be manual (using the hands to stimulate genitals), oral (using the mouth to stimulate genitals), rubbing (rubbing parts of the body or genitals against a partner's genitals), vibratory (using vibratory stimulation to stimulate genitals), or penetrative (penetrating the vagina or rectum for sexual pleasure). Needs in terms of erectile hardness vary greatly depending on which types of sex you want to have with a partner.

Intimacy is communication on all levels, moving towards deeper communication and understanding with a partner (Hatfield, 1982). Sex and intimacy often occur simultaneously, but they are two dis-

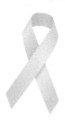

tinct concepts, and goals may pertain to one or both of these concepts. After prostate cancer treatment, you and your partner may find that you need deeper communication and understanding, and that involves intimacy (even without sexual relations). Intimacy brings closeness. This is important because one of the challenges of dealing with a cancer diagnosis is the potential for isolation between a man and his partner. Affection and physical touch may also be reassuring and play an important role in a deeper connection with a partner. Your thoughts and goals in terms of sex may vary greatly as you navigate through

All medical treatments have positive and negative effects, and prostate cancer treatments are no different.

prostate cancer diagnosis, treatment, and recovery. Even though sex may not be one of the most important things on a man's mind when first diagnosed with prostate cancer, it is likely to become a weighty concern.

Treatment Concerns

Prostate cancer is the most commonly diagnosed non-skin cancer in men, but early-stage prostate cancer is generally very survivable with treatment. There are several treatments for prostate cancer including surgery (prostate removal), radiation therapy (seed implants or external beam), hormonal therapy (negating or decreasing testosterone levels through androgen deprivation), and active surveillance (carefully monitoring prostate cancer progression). The most common treatment for early prostate cancer in younger, healthy men over the past several decades is surgery (prostatectomy [prostate removal]).

The concern for many men is that prostate cancer treatment is not without side effects, the most common being sexual dysfunction and urinary problems. All medical treatments have positive and negative effects, and prostate cancer treatments are no different. Even active surveillance can have some negative effects because leaving prostate cancer in the body can cause apprehension. For many men, quality of life after prostate cancer treatment is their greatest concern. Unfortunately, the negative effects of prostate cancer treatment can impact quality of life.

Erectile Dysfunction

Erectile dysfunction (ED) is the most common problem after removal of the prostate (surgery), radiation therapy, and androgen deprivation therapy. The National Institutes of Health (NIH) defines erectile dysfunction as the "inability to attain and/or maintain a penile erection sufficient for satisfactory sexual performance" (NIH Consensus Development Panel on Impotence, 1993) and this definition was subsequently accepted by the World Health Organization and the International Consultation on Urologic Disease (Jardin et al., 2000). Men experiencing ED after prostate treatment have trouble getting and/or keeping erections hard enough for penetrative types of sexual activity. ED can be caused by any disease process that impacts nervous conduction and/or blood flow such as diabetes, high blood pressure, heart disease, high cholesterol, obesity, head/neck/back disorders, or stroke (to name a few). ED can also be caused by surgery or radiation that impacts nervous conduction or blood flow necessary for erections.

Prevalence of ED in men after prostatectomy has been explored in many studies and has been reported to be as high as 78%-88% (Korfage et al., 2005; Penson et al., 2008). Erectile dysfunction in men who undergo radiation therapy is equally prevalent when compared to the prevalence of men with ED after prostate removal (surgery) (Yarbro & Ferrans, 1998). Erectile dysfunction has a negative impact on quality of life or life satisfaction (Potosky et al., 2004). Sexual function remains important to many men, who often continue to be interested in sex in the later decades of life (Frankel et al., 1998; Mul-

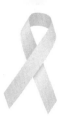

ligan & Moss, 1991). In light of the high survival rates associated with prostate cancer, issues impacting quality of life, such as ED, need to be addressed and treated in those men who are upset by their inability to get and keep erections.

Normal Erections

Men get erections every single day. The penis is erect approximately 3 out of every 24 hours, primarily during deep rapid eye movement (REM) sleep at night. A man experiences approximately 4-6 erections every night. When a man thinks sexual thoughts or his penis is stimulated or both, that information is synthesized in the frontal lobe of the brain. The message travels down the spine to the peripheral nerves. The peripheral nerves wrap around the prostate and go to the penis. In the penis, the nerve impulse activates chemicals in the penis which tell the blood vessels to dilate. The penis becomes engorged with blood, making it erect.

Every night a man's penis gets a workout with the smooth muscles around the blood vessels expanding and contracting to let more blood in the penis when it is erect and allowing less blood in the penis when it is flaccid. This is like pushups for the penis! The muscles around the penis literally get a workout from relaxation and contraction around the blood vessels. The increased blood flow associated with nighttime erections helps to keep the tissue of the penis healthy and normal. After prostate removal or radiation of the prostate, the nerves for erections are traumatized and do not conduct properly. Sometimes it is necessary to remove these nerves during surgery. This happens when the cancer has grown close to where the nerves lie on the back of the prostate. If the nerves are removed, they cannot conduct impulses. Not only can conduction be compromised from the dissection of these nerves away from the prostate or radiation of the nerves, but the chemicals in the penis that tell the muscles to dilate may also be diminished. The cavernosal nerve is a source of synthesis for nitric oxide, which is one of the most important chemicals in the penis that helps blood vessels dilate (Carrier et al., 1995). This lack of nerve conduction can lead to less blood flow to the penis in terms of penile engorgement and can change the structure of the penis and lead to diminished muscle function.

Discovery and Learning

It is important to understand some things about research. Research is about discovery and learning new information about people and the treatments they are undergoing. There is a great deal of research presented in this book and the references that correspond with that research. The research presented here provides some information about penile rehabilitation. The goal of penile rehabilitation is to preserve maximum erectile function and length, and increase blood flow, which is important to proper function of the smooth muscles of the penis.

Not all research is equally relevant. The best information gleaned from research comes from the highest levels of scientific study. These studies are typically placebo controlled (the treatment is compared to a similar looking but fake treatment), randomized (participants are randomly assigned to the treatment or placebo portions of the study), and blinded (participants do not know if they are receiving the treatment or not). Outcomes of studies are stronger if the researchers can compare a newer treatment to something that looks the same, but is not the real treatment (a placebo). Even when researchers conduct a randomized blinded placebo-controlled trial, the design may have flaws; therefore, it is important to examine the study carefully to understand the value of the information discovered. Randomized blinded placebo-controlled studies are expensive, and they are not always fea-

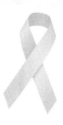
sible. Sometimes scientists compare different types of treatments to each other, which can also be helpful. It is not always possible to have a comparative or placebo treatment because it would not be ethical for a scientist to withhold a treatment proven to be effective from patients in a control group. One example of a treatment that can't be studied in a placebo-controlled blinded study is the vacuum device. It would be impossible to use a placebo device because the real device would be readily apparent and have working suction.

Another important factor to think about when reviewing the strength of a study is the size of the sample (the number of participants). Larger numbers of participants and a wide variety of participants from various places (rather than one institution) also strengthen the findings of a study. Penile rehabilitation research with medications and vacuum devices is newer and more research needs to be done. Some of the studies did not use comparative groups and are relatively small in sample size. Although it is valuable and important to do studies of all sizes in all settings, it is always important to keep the findings in context.

Many references are provided in this book to give you the information you need to learn more about the studies. In fact, you may even find some newer research about erectile dysfunction treatment and penile rehabilitation that has emerged since this book was published. It is important to promote blood flow to the penis after treatment for prostate cancer to preserve maximal erectile function. There is still much research to be done in the area of sexual dysfunction after prostate cancer treatment. However, new research shows that medical treatments for ED may have promise in terms of preserving maximal penile erection function after prostate cancer treatment. It is my hope this book will provide the knowledge and inspiration needed for you to reclaim sex and intimacy after prostate cancer.

Chapter 2
Prostatectomy, Radiation Therapy, and Androgen Deprivation Therapy

One question asked frequently in terms of prostate cancer is whether it is necessary to treat every prostate cancer. Some prostate cancers are aggressive and will grow quickly, while others are indolent (slow to develop) and grow very slowly. Slow-growing prostate cancers may not require treatment, but rather active surveillance to monitor progression carefully. A man can live a full, productive life with prostate cancer and it may not lead to major problems. However, not every man is comfortable with watching, rather than treating, his prostate cancer. The risk with not treating prostate cancer is that it may spread outside the prostate, making it more difficult to treat. Yet, as experts determine better ways to monitor prostate cancer, some men may feel more comfortable actively monitoring prostate cancer rather than treating it.

Surgery

Removal of the prostate (prostatectomy) is typically done as a primary therapy with a goal of getting rid of the cancer completely. Removal of the prostate continues to be a gold standard treatment option for prostate cancer against which all other treatment options are measured (Zippe et al., 2001). The reason is surgery has been done longer than any other treatment, and, therefore, we know more about it than any other treatment. This does not mean surgery is the best choice for you, but it means we know a lot about this option because it has been performed for many years.

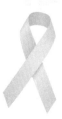

In an effort to preserve erectile function after prostatectomy, nerve-sparing techniques have been developed to save the nerves involved in erectile function (Walsh & Mostwin, 1984). Nerves run along the back side of the prostate and must be dissected off it in order to remove the prostate. Despite advanced techniques in nerve sparing, erectile dysfunction remains a problem for the majority of men following radical prostatectomy (Penson et al., 2005; Walsh, Marschke, Ricker, & Burnett, 2000). Researchers continue to seek better techniques to improve erectile function after radical prostatectomy and to minimize damage to the nerves responsible for erections.

...as experts determine better ways to monitor prostate cancer, some men may feel more comfortable actively monitoring prostate cancer rather than treating it.

The most predominant technique of recent years to minimize side effects of prostate removal is robotic radical prostatectomy. Robotic-assisted prostatectomy employs minimally invasive surgical techniques using a laparoscope (a long tube that provides magnified visualization and access through which to perform procedures) and approximately five to six small ports of entry to remove the prostate rather than the traditional open method of prostatectomy (El-Hakim & Tweari, 2004). The surgeon sits at a command console and uses hand controls that allow each of his movements to be translated into movements with the robotic instruments within the body while simultaneously filtering tremors, scaling movement to size, and providing full range of motion through the instruments within the body. The cameras in the laparoscope provide a three-dimensional magnified image for the surgeon. In terms of erectile function, the hope is the robotic-assisted method will provide a more precise surgical technique, less manipulation, and better visualization of the nerves for erectile function during prostate removal.

Despite the newer techniques of robotic prostatectomy, ED continues to be the most common negative long-term outcome after robotic radical prostatectomy (Menon et al., 2005). In the hands of an experienced surgeon, potency rates are comparable for robotic and open radical prostatectomy (Menon et al., 2005; Menon et al., 2007; Penson et al., 2008). The majority of men report problems with erection immediately following the procedure and some do not regain the function they had preoperatively. Regardless of the type of prostate removal you have undergone, it takes an average of 2 years for nerves to recover after surgery. The nerves may recover sooner, but the average is 2 years, so don't get discouraged if your erection is returning slowly.

Regardless of the type of prostate removal you have undergone, it takes an average of 2 years for nerves to recover after surgery.

Radiation

Radiation therapy is another common treatment for prostate cancer. Although radiation is directed toward the prostate with external beam radiation, or from within the prostate with brachytherapy (seed implants), the nerves for erections which run along the posterior side of the prostate can be traumatized and damaged from radiation exposure. The quest continues to improve delivery of radiation to the prostate in the most precise manner to minimize exposure to the nerves responsible for erections, but, currently, ED is the most common long-term side effect from radiation therapy. The full impact of radiation on the penis is usually not completely determined until about 12 or more months after treatment. The negative effects on erections worsen over time as changes continue to take place within

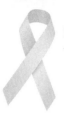

the body after radiation therapy. Diminished erectile function occurs slowly over time after radiation therapy is complete.

Androgen Deprivation

Androgen deprivation therapy may be used in combination with other treatments or alone. The goal of androgen deprivation therapy is to suppress testosterone levels and thereby decrease prostate cancer growth. The main sexual side effects of this treatment are decreased sex drive and erectile dysfunction. A decreased sex drive may also diminish motivation for dealing with the added burden of ED treatments needed for sexual relations.

Chapter 3
Orgasms: Sex without Erections

This may seem like a very strange topic and even may appear to be an oxymoron, but it is not. If you have not discovered it yet, most men *can* have a climax/orgasm without an erection.

Erections are wired separately through the nervous system from the ability to climax. The majority of men still experience a climax/orgasm sensation after prostate cancer treatment especially with nerve-sparing techniques. You will likely not ejaculate during climax after prostate cancer treatment because the prostate and nearby glands play a crucial role in ejaculation. Some men say the orgasm is similar to the ones they had prior to surgery (even without the fluid ejaculate). Other men say the orgasms are not as intense and feel less enjoyable, but they still climax. Surprisingly, some men report that orgasms are better after prostate removal or treatment. The large majority of men continue to enjoy orgasms after prostate cancer treatment. Some men report a degree of pain with orgasms in the first month or two after surgery, but this typically does not persist and most men eventually will enjoy orgasms after prostate cancer treatment. If you continue to have pain with climax, it is important to let your health care provider know because this problem may be resolved with medications.

The majority of women climax from clitoral stimulation, so the good news is that your female partners can climax with or without your erection. Women typically take four times longer than men to reach

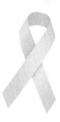

climax, so foreplay must focus on stimulation that is most pleasing to a female partner.

Some couples choose to enjoy non-penetrative sex such as manual or oral stimulation. Mutual masturbation can be enjoyable or you can stimulate each other through a variety of other ways. The important thing is to discover what each of you enjoys and explore all options for stimulation, cuddling, and climaxing together. Some couples may even choose not to be sexual together and, if both agree that this is acceptable, this is a perfectly valid choice. Men and women can climax from many types of stimulation, so determine what you

Don't let your affection for your partner suffer because of lack of communication or misconceptions.

and your partner are most comfortable with and explore those options. Sometimes when men or women have trouble climaxing, vibratory stimulation can make a difference. Although most women climax from clitoral stimulation and men from penile stimulation, vibratory stimulation may also be enjoyable in other areas of the body such as below the scrotum in men or around the rectum in men and women. Sample and explore the options together.

Some couples do not communicate about sex, and this can be a big problem when either of them worry about the other person's expectations, needs, or feelings, but don't clarify or talk about those issues. Some men and women stop being affectionate because they are afraid the other person might feel uncomfortable with anything that may lead to sex or intimacy. Physical affection can be very important in terms of intimacy and closeness, and there is no reason to stop kissing, holding hands, embracing, and touching each other. This physical affection can make your partner feel he or she is still attractive and can be very important in terms of self-esteem, image, and confidence. Talking about being affectionate and the fact that affection is not necessarily an indication of the need for sex can relieve anxiety and stress. Sex is different after prostate cancer and communication can be key in helping with this important change. Don't let your affection for your partner suffer because of lack of communication or misconceptions.

> *Sex is different after prostate cancer and communication can be key in helping with this important change.*

Orgasm and Urine Leakage

You may leak urine during sexual activity, particularly with orgasms. This is not that uncommon, even if you never leak urine any other time. Leakage is not unusual and not problematic because urine is sterile and not harmful. If urinary leakage bothers you or your partner, consider wearing a condom to prevent transfer of urine. This is unnecessary from a hygienic point of view, but some men and women may prefer this approach. Sometimes it can be helpful to empty the bladder immediately before sex. This may decrease urine leakage with orgasm. If this problem persists, consult your urology health care provider for advice.

Chapter 4
Penile Shrinkage

Some men have described shrinkage of their penis after radical prostatectomy. You may or may not have noticed shrinkage of the flaccid penis after prostate removal. Penile shrinkage has been documented in several studies (Kohler et al., 2007; Raina et al., 2006). Penile shrinkage may be related to several factors. Unchallenged muscle tone within the penis after removal of the prostate may cause some shrinkage. The penis is primarily a muscle and those muscles can shrink. When your penis is full of blood, the smooth muscles around the penis are relaxed; when your penis goes back to the soft/flaccid state,

The vacuum device may be of benefit for stretching the tissue of the penis and filling the penis with blood.

the muscles are contracted around the blood vessels. So if the muscles that surround the blood vessels are no longer contracting and relaxing with nighttime erections, the muscles of the penis are no longer getting a workout, muscle mass can diminish, and the penis can shrink. The flaccid penis seems to disappear up into the body. This diminished flaccid penis size can be upsetting for some men.

The vacuum device may be of benefit for stretching the tissue of the penis and filling the penis with blood. Men who used the vacuum device daily for a minimum of 10 minutes had less penile shrinkage and reported better erections. Maintaining flaccid penile length may occur with regular daily use of the vacuum device (Kohler et al., 2007). This will be discussed in detail in the treatment section of this book.

Chapter 5

Overview of Treatment of Erectile Dysfunction and Penile Rehabilitation after Prostate Treatment

The goal of erectile dysfunction treatment after prostate treatment is an erection sufficient for sexual relations. Although you may come across some incredible claims about treatments with herbal remedies, in general these medications do not work as well as the U.S. Food and Drug Administration-approved treatments discussed in this book. Some herbal treatments such as ginseng and yohimbine have had limited research showing a degree of efficacy. The problem is they generally do not work as well as other treatments discussed here and they do have side effects. If a purported treatment is as safe and effective as the current approved treatments, it should undergo the same rigorous research testing as the current approved options. Some men have spent a lot of money on these herbal treatments, which are not recommended by most experts in the field of sexual dysfunction.

There are four well-established medical treatment options for ED and each option has also been utilized for penile rehabilitation in men after prostatectomy.

There are four well-established medical treatment options for ED and each option has also been utilized for penile rehabilitation in men after prostatectomy. Initial research for each treatment option shows promise for helping to preserve erectile function. The goal of penile rehabilitation after prostate cancer treatment is to maximize erectile

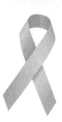

function recovery through the use of available medications and devices for treating erectile dysfunction. In terms of penile rehabilitation, the goal is to preserve pretreatment erectile function by promoting blood flow and oxygenation to the penis during the period of neuropraxia (erectile nerve dysfunction).

Each treatment must be evaluated and understood so you can make an educated and informed decision.

The first options are noninvasive and involve venous occlusive devices to keep blood in the penis during intercourse. They include the venous constriction device Venoseal® and the vacuum constriction device. The second option includes all oral phosphodiesterase type 5 (PDE-5) inhibitors such as Viagra® (sildenefil), Levitra® (vardenafil), Cialis® (tadalafil), and Stendra™ (avanafil). The third option is the urethral suppository, MUSE® (alprostadil). The fourth option is penile injections. The final option for treating ED (not for penile rehabilitation) is the surgical penile implant.

The Best Treatment for You

The ultimate question is how to determine which treatment is best for you and what treatment will provide the best erectile function recovery. There is currently insufficient research available to provide clear guidance; therefore, treatment selection is driven by your preference. Each treatment must be evaluated and understood so you can make an educated and informed decision. Each treatment has advantages and disadvantages. The pros and cons are presented in Table 1. Each treatment is described in detail in the following chapters.

It is important to keep in mind that different patients have different motivation levels in terms of sexual function and that motivational

Table 1.
Advantages and Disadvantages of ED Treatments

Treatment	Pros	Cons
Oral PDE-5 Inhibitors (pills)	Quick and easy to administer Discreet Suitable for travel	Poor efficacy rate in men after prostatectomy Side effects possible (headache, nasal congestion, flushing, stomach upset) Costly
Venous Constriction Devices (Venoseal and the Vacuum Constriction Device)	Noninvasive High efficacy rates Fairly quick and easy after "mastered" Suitable for travel May be incorporated into foreplay One-time cost	Cumbersome and awkward Messy Time consuming Penis may feel cool to touch and appear pink/purple Penis is wobbly at the base Challenges and comfort of wearing tension rings during sex May have side effects of bruising, pain, or discomfort
Intraurethral Suppository (MUSE)	Simple to use Less invasive than injections	Doesn't work in majority of men Side effects may occur (pain, burning, hypotension, increased heart rate, dizziness, and lightheadedness) Some patients uncomfortable with putting medication in urethra Expensive
Penile Injections	High efficacy rates Reliable treatment No tension ring needed Erection usually lasts about 60 minutes	Invasiveness: Need to inject the penis each time for erections Side effects possible (pain, bruising, bleeding, priapism, and Peyronie's disease) Need to refrigerate some medications Comfort level with self-injecting and the hassle of doing this procedure FDA-approved injections costly, but may be covered by insurance; trimix and bimix are much less expensive Some injectables must be refrigerated making travel challenging
Penile Implant	High efficacy rate High satisfaction rates No travel issues	Permanent Side effects (pain, infection, mechanical failure, and erosion of the device through the skin) Surgically invasive procedure Surgery is expensive

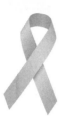
levels may also change over time. Your motivation for sex and intimacy is probably different than some other men. In one study, as many as half of patients (650 men) with ED after prostate cancer treatment reported indifference about erectile dysfunction, yet the use of at least one erection treatment aid was an independent determinant of more favorable sexual health related quality of life (Miller et al., 2006). Therefore, treating ED may improve life satisfaction for some men.

Treating ED may improve life satisfaction for some men.

Even though not everybody is concerned with sexual function, research continues to show that regular improved blood flow to the penis through medical treatments such as oral medications, vacuum device, intraurethral suppository, and/or the penile injections may improve a man's erectile function. Without regular blood flow to the penis, the penis may shrink and damage may occur to the penile tissue, further jeopardizing erectile function. Getting blood into the penis on a regular basis can be very important after prostate cancer treatment.

Chapter 6
Constriction Devices

Noninvasive options are used on the penis itself to provide erections sufficient for intercourse. Men have been putting tight bands and rings around their penis for many decades to help keep it hard during intercourse. There are many different tension loops and rings designed to help hold the blood in the penis advertised on the Internet and available in stores. The important safety feature that needs to be present on any ring or band is a mechanism to remove or release the tension after sex. Some of the hard rings without a release may actually get stuck on the penis, trapping the blood in the penis. No ring or band should be worn for longer than 30 minutes. It is essential to be able to release or stretch the band or ring to remove it from around the penis.

One such constriction device is Venoseal® (see Figure 1) which consists of an adjustable elastic loop that is placed and tightened around the base of the penis. This adjustable band is used to maintain blood within the penis during sexual relations and should not be worn for more than 30 minutes at a time. The Venoseal band is most helpful for men who get, but cannot keep, an erection since it will not make the penis much harder, but rather is designed to decrease blood flow back into the body by trapping the blood inside the erect penis. The advantages to the Venoseal band are that it is completely noninvasive and very simple to use. The Venoseal band costs about $25 and it is compact for travel. The disadvantages are that the tension band must be worn during sexual relations to maintain the erection and it may be uncomfortable as the elastic can catch or pull on pubic hair.

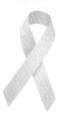
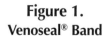

Figure 1.
Venoseal® Band

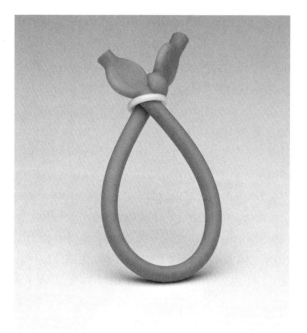

Reprinted with permission from Actient Pharmaceuticals/TIMM
Medical Technologies.

The vacuum constriction device is the second-most commonly prescribed treatment for erectile dysfunction. The vacuum constriction
device (see Figures 2 & 3) consists of a pump attached to a plastic
air-tight cylinder and a tension/constriction ring to maintain the erection. To use the device the penis is placed into the open end of the
cylinder that already has a previously applied tension ring at the
edge of the open end of the cylinder. The pump is on the opposite
end and when the device is placed against the body with the penis
inside, suction occurs from the negative pressure and blood is pulled
into the penis. The tension ring is applied to maintain the erection

Figure 2.
Osbon Erec-Aid® Esteem® Manual and Automatic Vacuum Therapy Systems

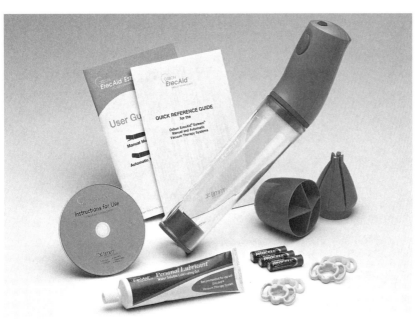

Reprinted with permission from Actient Pharmaceuticals/TIMM Medical Technologies.

during sex. The vacuum device works for most men if they are trained properly on its use. Efficacy of the vacuum constriction device, in terms of creating an erection sufficient for intercourse, has been reported as high as 87%-92%, regardless of the reason for the erectile dysfunction (Turner et al., 1991; Witherington, 1989). Long-term results of the device ranges from 50%-64% after 2 years (Cookson & Nadig, 1993). Success with the vacuum device is dependent on proper training since it can be tricky to apply and use. There are some very important tips for using the device which are outlined at the end of this chapter.

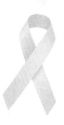

Figure 3.
SomaTherapy–ED®

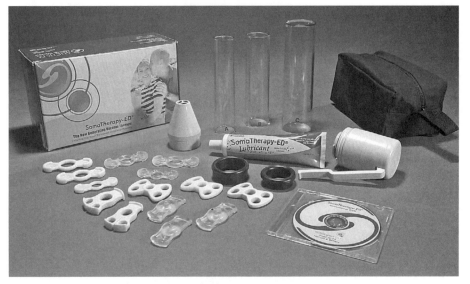

Reprinted with permission from Augusta Medical Systems.

Advantages of the vacuum device identified by patients in one study were that it was reliable, noninvasive, fairly quick and easy to use after practice, suitable for travel, and could add to the sexual experience if the couple is amiable to introducing the vacuum device into foreplay (Soderdahl, Thrasher, & Hansberry, 1997). In my clinical practice, with over a thousand men using the vacuum device, I can assure you it works. If used carefully, side effects are minimal, and this is what men like about this treatment. In addition, the cost is covered by most insurance providers including Medicare.

Disadvantages identified by patients include the fact that it is bulky, messy with the water-soluble gel, time consuming, the penis had a cool feeling to touch and was "hinged" or wobbly at the base, and that it detracted from the romance of the sexual situation (Soderdahl et al., 1997). In my practice, patients often express displeasure with the quality of an erection that feels unnatural and having to wear the tension ring during sex. The vacuum device is contraindicated for men with a history of priapism (persistent abnormal erection), sickle cell anemia, or certain bleeding disorders. In a comparison study with penile injections, both therapies were effective, but the dropout rates were much higher for penile injections versus the vacuum device (60% vs. 20%) (Turner et al., 1992). In men who failed to respond to intracavernosal injection therapy, 71% attained adequate rigid erections with the vacuum device (Gould, Switters, Broberick, & de-VereWhite, 1992). The vacuum device costs approximately $450-$550 and is covered by most insurance providers. The vacuum device requires one-on-one training with an expert provider and men need to utilize the treatment daily in the beginning to master it. The vacuum device is in no way discreet, and this may be an important factor for men who are not in a committed, understanding relationship.

The vacuum constriction device can also be used in conjunction with oral agents (PDE-5 inhibitors), which have been shown to increase efficacy and satisfaction (Chen, Sofer, Kaver, Matzkin, & Greenstein, 2004). Remember, the stronger the erection when put into the vacuum device, the easier it will be to get the penis to fill with blood and become hard enough for penetration. The oral pills may create a fairly natural partial erection and that can be put into the pump and brought to a complete erection. This is especially important for penile rehabilitation since the goal is to get as much oxygen-rich arterial blood into the penis as possible.

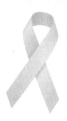

Penile Rehabilitation with the Vacuum Constriction Device

Some studies offer promising results for the use of the vacuum device for penile rehabilitation. Regular use of the vacuum device may improve return of spontaneous erections after prostate cancer treatment and may minimize penile shrinkage (Kohler et al., 2007; Raina et al., 2006). The combination of an oral agent and the vacuum device resulted in 30% of post-prostatectomy men reporting return of spontaneous erections and reports of improved satisfaction over therapy with either sildenafil or the vacuum device alone (Raina, Agarwal, Allamaneni, Lakin, & Zippe, 2005).

It is unclear exactly how much and how often the vacuum device should be used. In studies, the device was used for approximately 10 minutes a day, pumping up the penis several times, allowing it to sit inside the vacuum device full of blood for a few minutes, then releasing the suction and starting over. No tension rings were applied to the penis during daily rehabilitation, but the penis was filled with blood and kept erect inside the device for a few minutes at a time. These studies had a relatively small number of participants and further research is needed to determine the role of the vacuum device for penile rehabilitation. Although research is limited and ongoing, the use of the vacuum device in combination with oral agents for penile rehabilitation appears promising.

Arterial blood is crucial to bringing oxygenated blood to the tissue of the penis. That is why it is important to get as much arterial blood into the penis prior to putting it into the vacuum pump, since the device will pull both arterial and venous blood into the penis. Remember, the ring is not used during daily penile rehabilitation. When used in conjunction with the vacuum device, oral agents must be taken at least 1 hour prior to using the vacuum device. The penis should be stimulated to bring as much oxygen-rich blood into the penis as possible prior to placing it in the vacuum device.

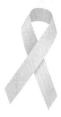

Keys to Success with the Vacuum Device

* Carefully read and follow the manufacturer's instructions for using your particular device as devices may vary.

* Shave or trim the hair around the penis so you get a good suction seal and the hair does not catch in the device.

* Always try and get your penis as full or hard as you can before placing it in the device.

* Lubricate the penis and the device.

* Make sure only the penis is placed in the device. The testicles and scrotum should not be in the device.

* Pump 2-3 times and stop. Let the penis fill with blood for a few seconds and then pump a few times and stop. Repeat this process until the penis is uniformly full. Do not over pump. You will feel pressure, but the process should not be painful. If you feel pain, hit the release button and pull the penis free of the device. Put the penis back in the device immediately and start over. You can also try a partial release by momentarily pressing the release button, but sometimes this may not work as well. You may need to do multiple releases to get the penis to fill properly to a full erection without pain.

* If the penis is getting too thick at the base and the blood is not flowing up to the head of the penis, hit the release button and pull the penis free of the device to completely break the suction. Immediately put the penis back inside the device and start pumping again. You can also try a partial release as noted above. Multiple partial or full releases may be needed to create an even, uniform erection that lifts off the bottom of the cylinder.

Keys to Success with the Vacuum Device *(continued)*

✳ If you continue to have trouble with extra tissue (skin) pulling into the pump around the base of the penis, you may need an insert for the opening of the vacuum device to keep the extra tissue from drawing into it. There are a variety of inserts available; contact the company that made your device for assistance. Some devices may have special rings that cover the end of the device with a hole in the middle to insert the penis. These rings may help keep other tissue from pulling into the device. It is important to work with trained professionals to help you obtain optimal erectile function from the vacuum constriction device.

✳ Take your time with the vacuum device. Do not use the tension rings until you have mastered pumping the penis up uniformly to a full erection without pain.

✳ Test the various tension rings to see which one will hold the erection best during sex. Preload the ring on the device before putting your penis in the device. When you have achieved a full erection inside the device, hold the device steady against your body with one hand (maintaining the suction), while creating a "V" with two fingers to push the ring off the device onto your erection. Do not break the suction seal prior to the ring going on your penis or the penis will not be hard enough for penetration. Never wear the ring longer than 30 minutes.

✳ If practicing or using the device for penile rehabilitation, do not use the rings! Only use the rings when you are trying to have sex. Work with the device for about 10 minutes each day, carefully pumping the penis to full as noted previously, letting it sit in the device erect for 2-4 minutes, and then releasing it. Repeat the process for 10 minutes a day.

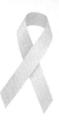

Notes from discussions with my provider/caregivers about the vacuum device.

_____

_____

_____

_____

_____

_____

_____

_____

_____

_____

_____

_____

_____

_____

_____

_____

_____

Chapter 7
Oral PDE-5 Inhibitors

Oral PDE-5 inhibitor agents (such as Viagra, Levitra, Cialis, and Stendra) continue to be the treatment of choice for men with erectile dysfunction, but, unfortunately, these agents have failure rates as high as 80% in men after prostatectomy (Baniel, Israilov, Segenreich, & Livne, 2001). This category of medications requires the nerves to work properly. Remember, even when the nerves for erections are spared, they do not always function well after surgery or radiation. As the preserved nerves recover after radical prostatectomy, the oral medications may become more effective. In randomized trials for patients complaining of ED after external beam radiation therapy, 55% and 57% of patients using Viagra and Cialis reported successful intercourse (Incrocci, Koper, Hop, & Slob, 2001; Incrocci, Slagter, Slob, & Hop, 2006).

Oral agents are taken by mouth approximately 1 hour (minimum) prior to sexual relations. Viagra, Levitra, and Cialis all take a minimum of 1-2 hours to maximize in the blood stream. Stendra takes 30-60 minutes to maximize. Oral agents work by inhibiting PDE-5, an enzyme that breaks down cyclic guanosine monophosphate (cGMP). Without the PDE-5 enzyme to diminish cGMP, the cGMP is increased. The cGMP is released during sexual arousal and is part of a group of chemical mediators that lead to smooth muscle relaxation and erections. Without stimulation through sexual thoughts or directly on the penis, the chemical is ineffective and the

Think of all the millions of men who use these pills and you can understand how important simplicity and discretion are to them.

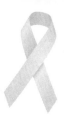

erections will not occur. So you must think sexual thoughts and/or have stimulation to the genitals for the erection to occur after taking the medication by mouth.

The greatest advantage to oral agents is that no other treatment is so simple to use, it does not require a man to step away from the sexual situation to administer the treatment, and it is discrete. Think of all the millions of men who use these pills and you can understand how important simplicity and discretion are to them. Traveling with the medication is not problematic since it does not need to be refrigerated. Oral PDE-5 inhibitors also are one of the least expensive pharmacological options (even though they may seem expensive to you). Prices vary among pharmacies, so shop for the cheapest price from a trusted, reputable pharmacy.

The biggest disadvantage to oral agents is that they are not always effective in producing an erection sufficient for sexual relations in men after prostate removal or radiation therapy. Oral agents will only work with preservation of the nerves responsible for erections because they rely on those nerves to activate the chemicals within the penis that will lead to increased blood flow and erections. If the nerves were not spared, oral agents will not be effective. Efficacy of Viagra (sildenafil) in men following radical prostatectomy varies greatly due to many different factors including pre-operative erectile function, extent of nerve sparing, and variations in definitions of erectile response and measurement of erectile function (Hatzimouratidis et al., 2009).

Common side effects include headache, facial flushing, nasal congestion, and stomach upset. These medications should not be used by men taking nitrates for chest pain (McMahon, Samali, & Johnson,

2000). Oral PDE-5 medications should be used cautiously in men who are taking alpha-adrenergic blocker medications (for enlarged prostate) because of the risk of sudden drop in blood pressure. Caution must also be used in men with renal impairment because the medications are excreted through the kidneys. If you have certain heart conditions, such as QT prolongation, oral PDE-5 inhibitors should be used cautiously and under medical supervision only. It is best to consult your personal primary care provider or cardiologist before taking these medications.

Penile Rehabilitation with Oral PDE-5 Inhibitors

Emerging research is conflicting in terms of early use of these medications for penile rehabilitation to promote better erectile function. The theory behind penile rehabilitation with these agents is that the drugs may provide improved blood flow and oxygenation to the penis, thereby improving function of the penis. Researchers evaluated erectile dysfunction in 76 men with normal pre-operative erectile function who underwent bilateral nerve-sparing radical prostatectomy (Padma-Nathan et al., 2003). The men took sildenafil 50-100 mg every night for 36 weeks beginning 4 weeks after surgery. Results showed that 27% of the men taking sildenafil versus 4% in the placebo group had a return of spontaneous normal erections. Although this is a small study, it did have a placebo comparison group, which improves the strength of these findings.

Emerging research is conflicting in terms of early use of these medications for penile rehabilitation to promote better erectile function.

Another study showed that men using 50-100 mg of sildenafil nightly had improved nocturnal erections compared with men treated with

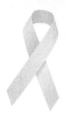

placebo (McCullough, Levine, & Padma-Nathan, 2008). The evidence for using oral medications such as sildenafil is further strengthened by a study comparing nightly use of sildenafil 25 mg with potency rates at 1 year of 86% versus 66% in the control group who took sildenafil on demand/as needed (Bannowsky, Schulze, van der Horst, Hautmann, & Junemann, 2008).

A study using Levitra (vardenafil) was very complicated in terms of design. The researchers found that taking the medication on demand (5-20 mg as-needed dosing) resulted in better erections than placebo or daily (5-10 mg) use. This has added to confusion about how often the medications should be taken, and optimal dosing of the oral medications for penile rehabilitation (Montorsi et al., 2008). The study is not without flaws, including the fact that participants in the on-demand group were able to titrate up to the highest dose as needed, while those in the daily dose group could not take more than 10 mg.

Correct education on the use of these medications will alleviate disappointment if full erections are not achieved.

Although research is conflicting about the efficacy and dosing of oral agents for penile rehabilitation, urology specialists around the world commonly use oral agents for penile rehabilitation (Tal, Teloken, & Mulhall, 2011). Providers may instruct the patient to take one of the oral agents (Viagra, Levitra, Cialis, or Stendra) either daily or three times a week for penile rehabilitation.

Aside from the lack of definitive research for using oral agents for penile rehabilitation, the drugs can be expensive and it may be financially challenging for patients to use the oral agents daily or three times a week. Men may have to pay for these medications out of pocket. Some insurance providers limit the number of treatments per month for erectile dysfunction. Men may not understand the benefit to taking these medications regularly when they are not producing a full erection suffi- cient for sex. Therefore, it is important for men to understand that although they may be using PDE-5 inhibitors for penile rehabili- tation after radical prostatectomy, these agents may not fully produce an erection suf- ficient for penetrative sex. Correct education on the use of these medications will alleviate

Men must understand the benefits of increased blood flow to the penis so they will continue to use the treatment for that specific purpose.

disappointment if full erections are not achieved. Men must under- stand the benefits of increased blood flow to the penis so they will continue to use the treatment for that specific purpose. In many cases, the medication will not produce an erection sufficient for sex, but any increase in blood flow increases the oxygen to the tissue and may help keep penile tissue healthy. These medications may also be used in combination with other treatment options such as the vac- uum device or MUSE®.

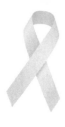

Keys to Success with Oral Medications

✳ Take the medication on an empty stomach or with a very low-fat diet since these medications are absorbed through the stomach and fat content in the stomach may slow absorption. Staxyn® (vardenafil) is a newer FDA-approved medication that dissolves on the tongue and is absorbed through the oral mucosa, not the stomach; therefore the food in the stomach is not a concern for effectiveness.

✳ Do not exceed the maximum dose of your medication.

✳ Wait at least 1-2 hours after taking the medication for the maximum medication effect. You must have sexual stimulation for these medications to work. Stendra (avanafil) is a newer medication that may reach peak effect in 30-45 minutes.

✳ These medications may decrease blood pressure slightly, so change positions slowly when taking these medications and lie down if you are dizzy or lightheaded. If you have persistent dizziness or lightheadedness, stop the medication and consult your health care provider.

✳ If you have visual acuity, peripheral vision, or hearing changes, stop the medication and seek medical help.

✳ Never take any of these medications if you take or carry medications with nitroglycerin. If you have chest pain and seek treatment, tell the providers that you take oral PDE-5 medications and when you last took a dose.

Keys to Success with Oral Medications

(continued)

✳ Some men have no side effects, but the most common ones for all these medications are headache, facial flushing, nasal stuffiness, and/or stomach upset. If you experience a headache from these medications, you might want to take acetaminophen or ibuprofen at the same time you take your erectile dysfunction medication. This may help alleviate the headache. If stomach upset is a problem, you might want to take the medication with a low-fat food like a cracker or pretzel. Viagra may cause color changes including blue colors around lights in some men. Cialis or Stendra may cause muscle aches in some men.

✳ You should only take these medications with a prescription from, and under the supervision of, a qualified prescriber.

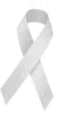

Notes from discussions with my provider/caregivers about my medications.

_____

_____

_____

_____

_____

_____

_____

_____

_____

_____

_____

_____

_____

_____

_____

_____

_____

Chapter 8
Intraurethral Alprostadil (MUSE®)

MUSE® (Medicated Urethral Suppository for Erections) is an intraurethral suppository of alprostadil (a prostaglandin) used for treating erectile dysfunction. After urination (when the urethra is wet) the MUSE (see Figures 4 & 5) applicator is inserted gently into the tip of the penis and passes about 1-2 inches down the urethra. The man depresses the button on the top of the applicator to release the MUSE into the urethra for absorption. After removing the applicator, the penis is rolled between the hands for a minimum of 10-30 seconds to dissolve the MUSE. MUSE is contraindicated in men with a hypersensitivity to alprostadil, men with an abnormally formed penis, or men who have conditions that would predispose them to priapism such as sickle cell anemia, leukemia, or tumors of the bone marrow. Caution must be used in patients with low blood pressure or a history of fainting since the medication may lower blood pressure and cause dizziness, lightheadedness, or fainting. Titrated dosages may start as low as 125-250 mcg and go up to 500-1,000 mcg.

When the medication was given to 384 men with or without nerve-sparing prostatectomy, 57% were able to have successful intercourse at least once at home as compared to 6.6% of the men receiving placebo (Costabile et al., 1998). Another research report indicated that regardless of the amount or ability to spare nerves during surgery, 55% of the patients achieved erections sufficient for intercourse with the treatment (Raina, Agarwal, Zaramo et al., 2005).

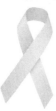

Figure 4.
Muse® Applicator and Parts

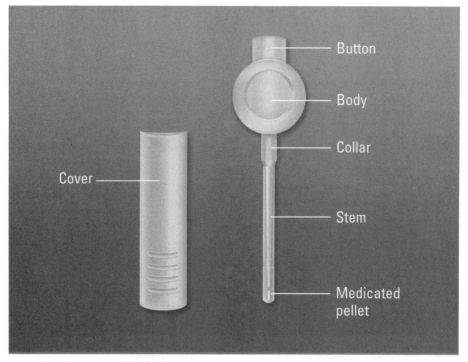

Reprinted with permission of Meda Pharmaceuticals, Inc.

One of the biggest issues with alprostadil/prostaglandin use in men after prostatectomy is pain. Since nerve endings are sensitized after prostatectomy or radiation, men may be more prone to the pain associated with alprostadil in the first year after treatment. In my experience with men post prostatectomy, the majority will experience pain with therapeutic doses of MUSE, which typically range from 500-1,000 mcg. Pain with these doses has also been described in the literature in anecdotal reports (Mulhall, 2008). Since pain is common after prostatectomy, the first dose of MUSE should be given in the

Figure 5.
Muse® Applicator Head in Hand and Used in Penis

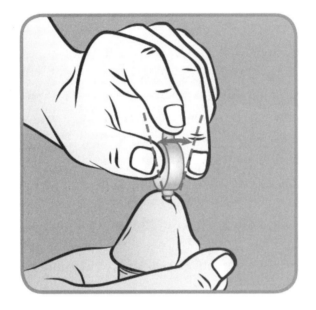

Reprinted with permission of Meda Pharmaceuticals, Inc.

physician's office or clinic, where blood pressure can be checked before and after administration. Low dosages of the drug should be used initially (Costabile et al., 1998; Raina, Pahlajani, Agarwal, & Zippe, 2008). That is why it is important to begin with sub-therapeutic doses of 125-250 mcg initially in men who have undergone prostate cancer surgery or radiation within the last year. The pain is dose dependent and may be lessened with a lower dose of the medication. If pain is an issue with this medication at lower doses, titrating upward to a dose that may produce an erection sufficient for sex is not an option because pain will intensify.

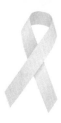

The advantage to MUSE is that it is simple to use and does not require a needle injection through the skin, as with the penile injections. MUSE can be unrefrigerated for up to 14 days at room temperatures of 30°-86° F. Therefore, it is easy to transport when traveling.

The disadvantages of MUSE are related to the fact that it does not always work to create an erection sufficient for sex in many men, it is expensive if not covered by insurance, and it may cause side effects. Adverse side effects most commonly reported are pain or burning, but may also include hypotension (low blood pressure), dizziness, lightheadedness, and fainting.

One of the biggest issues in men after prostatectomy is pain with prostaglandin use.

If the man scratches the urethra during insertion, bleeding may occur from the tip of the penis. MUSE costs about twice as much as the oral medications such as sildenafil or tadalafil.

MUSE can also be used in conjunction with a PDE-5 inhibitor in men after prostatectomy to increase efficacy. Check with your provider to make sure it is safe for you to use this combination of drugs before using them. Although research is limited, taking oral agents prior to instilling MUSE may be more effective than MUSE alone. One study included 23 men unsatisfied with sildenafil 100 mg alone who added MUSE 500 mcg (taking the sildenafil at least 1 hour prior) with 83% of the men reporting improved erectile rigidity (Nandipati, Raina, Agarwal, & Zippe, 2006; Raina et al., 2005). Of the men who had improvement in erection rigidity, they were rigid enough for vaginal penetration 80% of the time. In another study of 26 men who failed sildenafil and MUSE alone, men reported improved ability to have an erection sufficient for sex with the combination of sildenafil and MUSE together (Nehra, Blute, Barrett, & Moreland, 2002).

Although these reports are promising, more research is needed. In clinical practice, I have found that men may or may not get an erection sufficient for sex and if pain is intense enough, the medication will not be a good option for that man.

Penile Rehabilitation with Intraurethral Alprostadil (MUSE)

MUSE also may have a role in penile rehabilitation. There is emerging research on early intervention with MUSE after prostatectomy. The benefits of MUSE or injectable prostaglandin in terms of corporal oxygenation were reported as increasing oxygen saturation in the corpora (shaft) by 37%-57% despite marginal erectile response (Padmanaban & McCullough, 2006). In another study, researchers reported return of spontaneous erections after 6 months of tri-weekly MUSE in 39% of the men compared to 11% in the observational group (Raina, Agarwal, Nandipati, & Zippe, 2005). Another study of men with erectile dysfunction after prostatectomy compared early use of MUSE to delaying treatment and found that at 6 months 40% of men [38 men (a small study)] who continued using MUSE had return of natural erections sufficient for penetration (Raina, Agarwal, Nandipati et al., 2005). One study examined the possible mechanism of penile rehabilitation with MUSE and found that 125-250 mcg doses of alprostadil suppository improved corporal and glanular oxygen saturation levels, even in the absence of penile rigidity (McCullough, 2007). Further research is needed, but these studies provide evidence that MUSE may play a role in penile rehabilitation.

MUSE may play a role in penile rehabilitation.

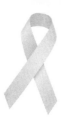

Keys to Success with MUSE

* MUSE should only be taken with a prescription from, and under the supervision of, a qualified prescriber.

* If using MUSE with an oral agent such as a PDE-5 inhibitor, take the oral agent at least 1 hour prior to MUSE. Check with your provider before trying this combination.

* If you experience pain when using MUSE, it may help to take whatever medication you take for a headache (acetaminophen, ibuprofen, or aspirin) about 30-45 minutes prior to administering MUSE.

* Check applicator to make sure the medication is present.

* Keep the penis upright during installation process and jiggle the applicator as you remove it to help drop the medication in the urethra.

* After administration, ensure the pellet was delivered by checking the applicator to make sure it is gone.

* Walk and stimulate the penis to promote increased blood flow to penis.

* A restrictive device, such as Venoseal, placed at the base of penis to decrease venous return from penis may be helpful and should not be in place more than 30 minutes.

* Lie down if dizzy, change positions slowly.

* Follow all directions in the MUSE patient education instructions/materials.

Notes from discussions with my provider/caregivers about MUSE.

_____

_____

_____

_____

_____

_____

_____

_____

_____

_____

_____

_____

_____

_____

_____

_____

_____

_____

_____

_____

Chapter 9
Intracavernosal Penile Injections

The man who is searching for a treatment option with a good track record in terms of efficacy, while providing a fairly natural feeling erection without a constriction ring, should consider penile injections. This therapy includes use of vasoactive medications injected into the side of the base of the penis to dilate the blood vessels of the penis and cause penile engorgement. Injections are more effective than intraurethral suppositories because the drug is delivered directly into the erectile cylinders of the penis rather than down the urethra (where it must travel across the urethra into the erectile cylinders). Commonly used injectable agents include monotherapy of prostaglandin in the form of Caverject®, Edex® (see Figure 6), off-label non-FDA approved compounded monotherapy of prostaglandin E1, or combination therapies using prostaglandin E1, papaverine, phentolamine, and/or atropine. Penile injections are contraindicated for men with a hypersensitivity to the medications; men with conditions that may lead to priapism including sickle cell anemia, multiple myeloma, and leukemia; and men with a penile implant or a severely deformed penis (Schwarz Pharma, 2004).

The advantage to penile injections is their effectiveness in producing fairly natural erections sufficient for intercourse. Penile injections are one of the most efficacious treatment options for men after prostatectomy with success rates reported as high as 85%-95% (Claro Jde et al., 2001; Dennis & McDougal, 1988). In our recent study of post-prostatectomy men, at 1 month after treatment with penile injections, 80% of the patients reported erectile function with the injections (Al-

Figure 6.
Edex® Dual Chamber Injection Device

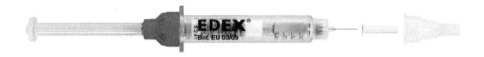

Reprinted with permission of Actient Pharmaceuticals/TIMM Medical Technologies.

baugh & Ferrans, 2010). At 3 months, 75% reported erectile function with the injections. Injections resulted in a significant improvement in erectile function as well as the self-esteem and satisfaction with sexual relationships. In previous research, patients stated the injections were quick and easy, not messy, and created a fairly natural erection without using tension rings to maintain the erection (Soderdahl et al., 1997).

Despite the excellent efficacy profile and the penile rehabilitation benefits of injections, some patients do not continue using this option and dropout rates are often as high as 55%-58% (Dennis & McDougal, 1988; Purvis, Egdetveit, & Christiansen, 1999). According to previous research, when comparing dropout rates for injections (not limited to prostatectomy patients, but including prostatectomy patients) with those for the vacuum device, the dropout rates for penile injections (60%) were three times greater than for the vacuum device (20%) (Turner et al., 1992). To increase success with penile injections, a man must be taught to inject the medication safely into the

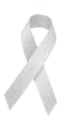

penis. This includes the ability to see the injection sites at the base of the penis, having the manual dexterity to inject safely, and the cognition to follow the instructions for self-injection. The first dose should be done in the physician's office or clinic under supervision to ensure safety with self-injection.

Disadvantages for injections identified by patients in previous research include the invasiveness of injections, problems with or fear of prolonged erections, pain, the need to refrigerate some of the medications, and the thought of the injections each time before sex (Albaugh & Ferrans, 2010; Soderdahl et al., 1997). Some injectables must be refrigerated and this can make travel with the medications challenging. Another disadvantage is that the FDA-approved versions of penile injections in the forms of Edex and Caverject are expensive. Compounded non-FDA approved, off-label penile injections are available from various compounding pharmacies and are less expensive (though they are often not covered by insurance prescription plans). Other patient-identified disadvantages for penile injections (not limited to men after prostatectomy) were inconvenience, lack of efficacy, cost, and side effects (Mulhall et al., 1999; Raina et al., 2003). These reasons for lack of use of injections were also identified in our recent pilot study with 20 men after radical prostatectomy. In terms of lack of efficacy, a total of seven men from this group (35%) were still struggling to find a consistent, effective dose with their injections approximately 3 months after beginning injections. Titrating injections can take time and require expert assistance from an experienced provider since a variety of injectable drugs have been studied and used since the 1980s. In our most recent pilot study with 20 men, we found that it can take one to eight dosage/medication changes before achieving efficacy (Albaugh & Ferrans, 2010).

Figure 7.
Intracaversonal Injection Sites Illustrated in Shaded Area

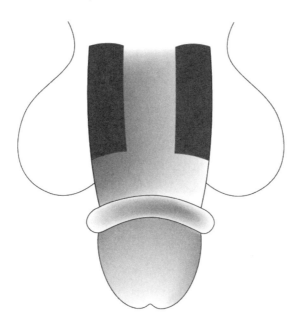

Reprinted with permission from Albaugh (2006).

Penile injection doses must be titrated carefully to a dose that creates an erection sufficient for sex (Albaugh, 2006). Injection therapy should be overseen by a urologic health care professional. The instructions provided here are general instructions to help you better understand penile injections, but these instructions are not meant to replace oversight by a trained health care professional.

Injections are given with a 0.5 or 1 ml syringe with 1/2 or 5/8 inch length, 27-30 gauge needle. The injection may be given anywhere from the base of the penis to two-thirds of the way down the penile shaft at the 10 o'clock and 2 o'clock locations on the upper side of the penis (see Figure 7). Typically, injections are rotated within that

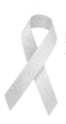

area and the side the injection is given is alternated with each injection to avoid scarring. Injection therapy can be given as a single agent (monotherapy) with alprostadil (prostaglandin E-1); a multi-agent mixture such as a trimixture of phentolamine, papaverine, and prostaglandin E1; a quadmixture of phentolamine, papaverine, prostaglandin E1, and atropine; or a bimixture of phentolamine and papaverine. Prostaglandin E1 can be compounded generically or as alprostadil either as Caverject or Edex. Lack of efficacy and cost have been described as reasons for using a combination of vasoactive agents instead of monotherapy with prostaglandin (Albaugh, 2006; Seyam, Mohamed, Akhras, & Rashwan, 2005). The FDA-approved medications are sometimes utilized because they are the most likely penile injectables to be covered by insurance.

Initial dosage should be determined by your health care provider. The initial dosing as recommended in the package insert for both Edex and Caverject is 2.5 mcg with a second dose of 2.5 mcg to be given if the initial dose is inadequate, but most clinics start dosing at the 5 mcg level. It is recommended the dose be increased by 5-10 mcg intervals at each attempt (a minimum of 24 hours apart) depending on the erectile response with each dose (up to a maximum dose of 40 mcg). Starting doses of compounded medications such as trimix or bimix will be determined by your health care provider. Typically trimix (papaverine 30 mg, phentolamine 1 mg, and prostaglandin E1 10 mcg) and bimix (papaverine 30 mg and phentolamine 1.5 mg) are started at a dose of 5-20 units (0.05-0.2 cc) in my clinic depending on the patient's age and concomitant problems for erectile dysfunction. The dose is increased by 1-5 units according to erection response during each test dose until a dose sufficient for sexual relations has been achieved. The maximum dose of trimix or bimix is usually no more than 100 units or 1 cc. Investigators have utilized dose volumes of trimix (papaverine 30 mg, phentolamine 1 mg, and prostaglandin 10 mcg per 1 cc) ranging from 0.18-1.0 cc in previous studies (Bennett, Carpenter, & Barada, 1991; Montorsi et al., 1997; Montorsi et al., 2002; Mulhall et al., 1999). If the test dose at home is inadequate, do not reinject more medication, but wait at least 24 hours for the next trial and then try a slightly higher dose.

Although it sounds very painful, men do not find the needlestick involved in penile injections to be painful.

The main concern with re-dosing or increasing the dose too quickly is priapism (an unbendable erection lasting for greater than 2-4 hours). Priapism is considered a medical emergency and must be resolved to avoid permanent damage to the penis. Priapism has been reported in as many as 11%-18.5% of men (Claro Jde et al., 2001; Porst, 1996). Priapism lasting 3-4 hours occurred in 4 of the 20 patients in our recent study, but the erection resolved spontaneously in all four men without needing to go to the emergency room. Some of the patients in our study struggled between taking enough medication to produce an erection sufficient for sexual relations and an erection that lasted too long (2-4 hours) (Albaugh & Ferrans, 2010).

A Scary Proposition

The thought of sticking a needle in the shaft of the penis is scary. Although it sounds very painful, men do not find the needlestick involved in penile injections to be painful. The pain is typically not related to needle insertion, but rather the side effect of the prostaglandin medication. In one of our studies (not limited to men after prostatectomy), we found that 40% of the 65 patients rated the needle insertion pain at 0 on a 0-10 verbal pain scale during their

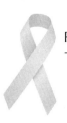

first office self-injection (Albaugh & Ferrans, 2009). For men who reported any pain from the needle insertion, the average pain rating was only 1.33 on a 1-10 verbal pain scale. We found a significantly larger proportion of post radical prostatectomy men experienced pain from the medication compared with men who had not undergone this procedure (51.9% vs. 23.7%) (Albaugh & Ferrans, 2009). In another study that was not limited to men after prostatectomy, pain from injected medication was reported in 29% of the patients using monotherapy with a prostaglandin product (Porst, Buvat, Meuleman, Michal, & Wagner, 1998). In our study of 20 men after prostatectomy, only about 25% of the men reported pain from the medication, but many of those men used trimix with lower doses of prostaglandin (Albaugh & Ferrans, 2010).

The thought of sticking a needle in the shaft of the penis is scary.

When pain is an issue for a man, lower dosages of prostaglandin in combination with other vasoactive injectable agents (papaverine and phentolamine) may be advisable. It has been reported that although the injections worked in the early months after prostatectomy, pain with prostaglandin was a significant issue and led to discontinuation in the majority of patients (Gontero et al., 2003). If necessary, prostaglandin can be eliminated altogether in patients who continue to have pain even at lower doses by using alternative vasoactive drugs such as a bimix solution of papaverine and phentolamine. Previous research (not limited to prostatectomy patients) has shown that switching to a trimix (papaverine/phentolamine/PGE1) or even a bimix (papaverine/phentolamine) combination is associated with lower incidence of pain (2.9% for trimix and 0 for bimix) (Baniel et al., 2000).

Another promising injectable agent currently under investigation in the United States is a combination of vasoactive intestinal polypeptide and phentolamine, which is currently undergoing Phase III clinical trials in the United States. Results from the manufacturer shows less incidence of pain (Gerstenberg, Metz, Ottesen, & Fahrenkrug, 1992; Sandhu et al., 1999; Shah, Dinsmore, Oakes, & Hackett, 2007).

Another side effect that may occur is bleeding and/or bruising. Less-common side effects include priapism and penile fibrosis/plaque formation. Priapism was discussed earlier. Peyronie's disease (curvature of the penis related to plaque formation) is not as common, but can be debilitating in terms of sexual activity. In terms of penile fibrosis/plaque/curvature in our recent pilot study, two (10%) patients reported a plaque or slight curve with injections. Rates of up to 14% of fibrosis/plaque/Peyronie's have been reported in the literature related to the penile injections (Schwarz Pharma, 2004). To minimize the risk of developing Peyronie's disease, it is important to rotate injection sites and hold pressure over injection sites (even if you do not see blood) for 5 minutes as directed in the prescribing information (Schwarz Pharma, 2004).

It is important to work closely with your health care provider to determine the best way for you to treat your erectile dysfunction and achieve penile rehabilitation.

Penile Rehabilitation with Intracavernosal Penile Injections

Regarding penile rehabilitation, injections were the first medical ED treatment to be used successfully for penile rehabilitation after prostatectomy to improve return of spontaneous erections (Montorsi et al., 1997). This was a small study, but it showed encouraging results. After 6 months the group receiving the penile injections had a

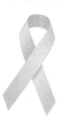

67% return of spontaneous erections sufficient for intercourse versus a 20% return of spontaneous erections for the control group. The researchers hypothesized the injections improved oxygenation to the tissue to enhance return of spontaneous erections.

In another study, 101 patients used prostaglandin E1 injections resulting in increased penile oxygen saturation 37%-57% (Padmanaban & McCullough, 2006). Another study reported that 56% (10 of 18 patients) who had used a combination of oral agents and injections of alprostadil had return of partial erections at approximately 6 months, but they still needed treatment to have sexual intercourse (Raina et al., 2008). The researchers also used trimix injections with four additional patients and reported that of the 22 total patients on either alprostadil or trimix, 50% had return of natural erections at 6 months. In another study using oral PDE-5 inhibitors for penile rehabilitation, patients who failed the oral agents were treated with intracavernosal injections (Mulhall, Land, Parker, Waters, & Flanigan, 2005). After 18 months, the men undergoing penile rehabilitation had a greater percentage of success engaging in intercourse unassisted by medication (52% vs. 19%). These were small studies, but they did have comparison groups.

A significant difficulty with penile rehabilitation using penile injections is convincing men to self-inject approximately 3 times a week, since injections are perceived as invasive and sometimes associated with pain in the early period after radical prostatectomy. Even with close observation and titration, pain was still a barrier identified by 4 of the 20 men in our study (Albaugh & Ferrans, 2010). Although researchers found that starting injections in the first month after surgery resulted in better erectile response, participants also reported more pain (Gontero et al., 2003).

In our recent pilot study with 20 patients, patients used the injections an average of four times per month (Albaugh & Ferrans, 2010). Despite agreeing to use the injections a minimum of at least four times a month, seven men did not use the injections even once per week. Not all men will use the injections regularly for penile rehabilitation. Some men using injections will use oral agents for penile rehabilitation on the days they are not using the injections, so they are regularly using either the oral pills or the injections. The injections and the pills may have a synergistic effect leading to priapism and, therefore, it is best to not take the pill within 24-36 hours of the injection. It is important to work closely with your health care provider on your injections to determine the safest and best way for you to treat your erectile dysfunction and achieve penile rehabilitation.

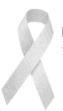

Keys to Successful Injections

* Please be very careful and follow all the written and verbal instructions you were given for your injections from your provider/caregivers.

* Do not inject more than one time in a 24-hour period or two to three times a week maximum regardless of whether or not you achieved an erection with the injections.

* Rotate the sites in the areas you were taught to inject.

* Press on the injection site for about 5 minutes after the injection with the fingers on one side of the penis pressing against the thumb on the other side of the penis.

* Follow all instructions if you experience a priapism (an unbendable erection for 2 or more hours). If you have questions about the instructions and/or if the erection persists after 2 hours, go to the emergency room with the instructions you were given.

* After 6-8 hours a prolonged erection (priapism) can cause permanent tissue damage and becomes more difficult to treat. Sometimes it helps to increase activity and move around to try and get the blood to move out of the penis (for example, some men will run up and down the steps a few times or jog in place). It may also help to lie on your back, allowing the blood to drain out of the penis. Sometimes a warm or cold pack may help resolve the erection, but if these things are not working, you need to do something further. If you have a priapism lasting 2 hours, some patients have found it helpful to take one of the following medications (these medications are used for other purposes, but have been used by patients outside the medication's primary indication as an antidote for a priapism):

Keys to Successful Injections
(continued)

- Pseudoephedrine (Sudafed®) 30 mg tablets (no prescription needed, but you must ask the pharmacist for this medication). Take one to two tablets by mouth. (Do not exceed 60 mg total unless your health care provider specifically told you to take more than 60 mg.) If you cannot take pseudoephedrine related to allergies, uncontrolled high blood pressure, heart problems, or any other reason, proceed to the emergency room for treatment (read the label information on the pseudoephedrine before taking it to see if you can safely take this medication). If the pseudoephedrine doesn't work after 1 hour, go to the emergency room for treatment.

- Terbutaline 5-10 mg may be taken orally to treat a priapism. This medication requires a prescription. If the medication does not work after 45 minutes, go to the emergency room.

✳ Do not inject into your penis when under the influence of alcohol or drugs.

✳ If you are having problems with injections, stop injecting and call your health care provider for further instructions. Injections must be done under the guidance of an expert provider.

✳ These instructions are in no way meant to substitute for expert one-on-one education with a qualified provider.

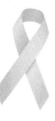

Notes from discussions with my provider/caregivers about penile injections.

_____

_____

_____

_____

_____

_____

_____

_____

_____

_____

_____

_____

_____

_____

_____

_____

_____

_____

_____

_____

Chapter 10
Penile Prosthesis

The penile prosthetic implant was one of the first treatments for erectile dysfunction. The implant is surgically placed within the penis within each corpora cavernosa (column of erectile tissue). The malleable implant was one of the first designs (see Figures 8 & 9) and is very simple to operate. The man bends the penis upward when he wants to have sexual relations and bends the penis out of the way when he is not sexually active. The malleable implant is always semi-erect so it does not ever become flaccid. Subsequent designs in protheses eliminated this disadvantage by creating an inflatable implant (see Figures 10-12) that utilizes a manual pump in the scrotum to draw fluid into the cylinders of the penile implant for inflation and a release mechanism to drain the fluid back into the abdominal reservoir. This implant more closely mimics the normal flaccid and erectile state, although the cylinders never completely deflate. Even when a man is flaccid the cylinders provide a little bit of length and girth in the penis.

Satisfaction rates with penile implants are high at approximately 83%-85%.

The advantage to a penile implant is that it is effective, more spontaneous, and patients are typically satisfied with this treatment. Satisfaction rates with penile implants are high at approximately 83%-85%. Complication rates, such as mechanical failure or infection, remain low at 6.4%-13.7% and 1.7%-1.8% respectively (Montague & Angermeier, 2000, 2003). Although penile prosthesis implantation makes the return of spontaneous erections impossible,

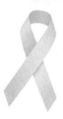

Figure 8.
Spectra™ Concealable Penile Prosthesis

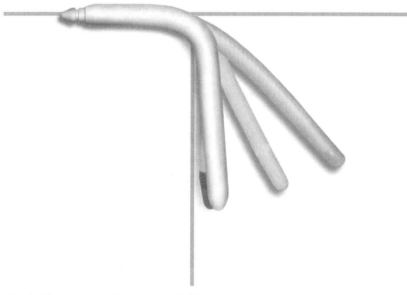

Reprinted with permission of American Medical Systems, Inc.

simultaneous implantation of a penile prosthesis at the time of prostatectomy has been associated with improvement in quality of life in patients (Ramsawh, Morgentaler, Covino, Barlow, & DeWolf, 2005). It is a reliable treatment, but because it is the most invasive treatment and surgery permanently alters the corpora cavernosa, preventing the use of other medical therapies, most patients considered it the final line of treatment after medical treatments have failed.

Figure 9.
AMS Spectra™ Prosthesis

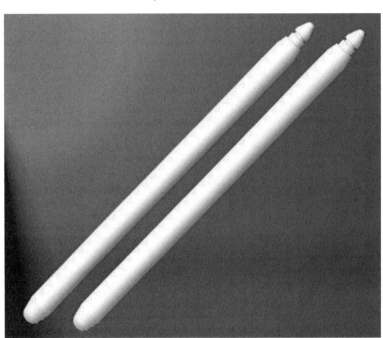

Reprinted with permission of American Medical Systems, Inc.

The patient who wants to undergo an implant must be a good candidate for surgery and needs to be prepared and accepting of the permanency of the implant option. Travel is not an issue since the prosthesis is implanted in the body. The prosthesis can be used at anytime and involves a one-time cost. The implant is an accepted treatment covered by most insurance plans.

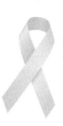

Figure 10.
AMS 700™ Series Inflatable Penile Implant

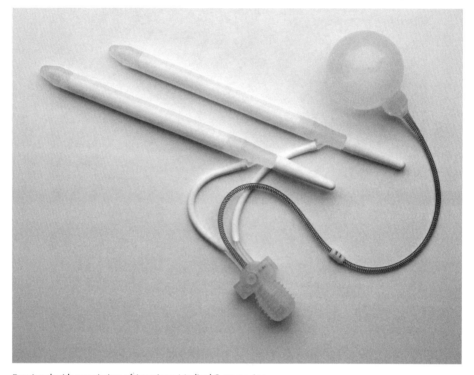

Reprinted with permission of American Medical Systems, Inc.

Disadvantages to the implant include pain after the procedure, and less commonly mechanical failure or infection (Montague & Anger-meier, 2003). The most common adverse effect of the implant is pain after the implant surgery that typically resolves a few weeks to a few months after surgery. The implant also involves the typical risks involved with any surgery. The penile implant surgery costs about $8,000-$12,000 (costs and insurance coverage may vary).

Figure 11.
Titan OTR® Inflatable Penile Prosthesis

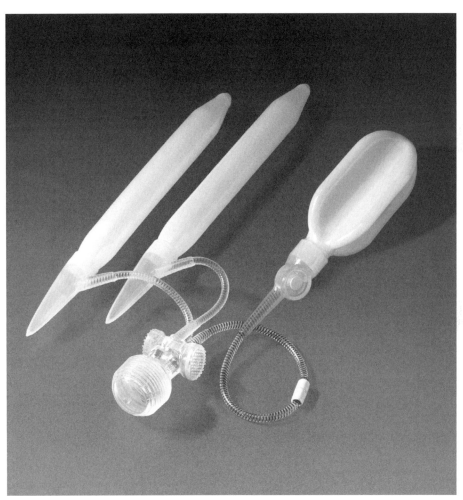

Reprinted with permission of Coloplast Corporation.

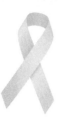

Figure 12.
Titan OTR® Inflatable Penile Prosthesis

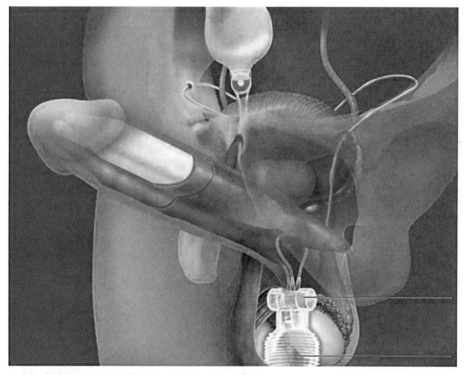

Reprinted with permission of Coloplast Corporation.

Keys for Success with the Penile Implant

✳ You should follow all the specific instructions from your caregivers. These keys outlined here are only meant to be basic guidelines.

✳ Some men may use the vacuum device daily for tissue stretching for about 10 minutes a day for several weeks before surgery as described in the vacuum constriction device section (without a tension ring) to stretch the penile tissue in preparation for penile implant.

✳ Immediately following surgery, you may need to wear snug-fitting jockey shorts or an athletic supporter (check with your surgeon).

✳ You may need to apply a cold pack to the groin area (on top of your jockey shorts or supporter) to decrease swelling and bruising for the first 24 hours. Do not put the cold pack directly on the skin, but be sure you have clothing or a towel between the skin and the cold pack. Often the penis and scrotum will swell (double in size) and become bruised despite using ice packs. You will be given pain medication to use as needed.

✳ Take showers or sponge baths for the first 7-10 days after your surgery. After 7-10 days, you may take warm baths, which might relieve the pain and soreness you may feel, especially after being up on your feet for a while. Apply antibiotic ointment to your incision twice a day or as directed by your provider, especially after showering or bathing. You may have a slight amount of drainage from the incision site, but if you notice persistent drainage, increasing redness, increasing pain or burning at the incision site, call your provider or seek medical help.

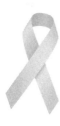

Keys for Success with the Penile Implant *(continued)*

✳ Take your medications as prescribed. You will be given an oral antibiotic that must be taken until the pills are gone.

✳ Do not have sexual intercourse for at least 6 weeks after your operation, or until your doctor tells you the surgical site has healed.

✳ At some point after surgery (within a few weeks), you will meet with your provider or the urology staff to inflate and deflate the inflatable prosthesis for the first time. They may have you practice inflating and deflating at regular intervals during the healing process, but follow the instructions of your provider carefully for the best outcome. You may have some pain for several weeks when inflating or deflating after surgery, but the pain will generally improve over time and as you become skilled at inflating and deflating the prosthesis.

✳ Watch for signs of infection:

- Fever

- Increasing pain

- Increasing swelling in the penis or scrotum

- Increasing drainage from penis or incision area (area that was cut)

- Inability to urinate

✳ If you notice any signs of infection or have any other problems, call your provider or go to an urgent care center or emergency room.

**Notes from discussions with my provider/caregivers
about penile prosthesis.**

_____

_____

_____

_____

_____

_____

_____

_____

_____

_____

_____

_____

_____

_____

_____

_____

_____

_____

Chapter 11
Urinary Incontinence

Urinary incontinence is an accidental loss of urine. Research reveals approximately 15% of men are incontinent up to 1 year following either radical prostatectomy or laparoscopic prostatectomy. It can take as long as 2 years for patients to regain continence (Jacobsen, Moore, Estey, & Voaklander, 2007; Sacco et al., 2006). Men treated for prostate cancer know that when the catheter comes out the leakage may begin. For many men, this leakage may resolve over the next year, but for some men the issue may last longer. During prostatectomy, part of the mechanisms that maintain the urine in the bladder are removed. As a result, the remaining pelvic floor muscles must work harder to maintain the urine in the bladder with activity, coughing, sneezing, and laughing. Men may also have a more urgent need to urinate and not be able to get to the bathroom before leakage occurs. If a man has had radiation therapy, he also may have problems with incontinence related to urinary urgency.

Incontinence can be treated successfully for the majority of men.

To help better understand urinary incontinence, this problem can be divided into different categories. Each type of incontinence is different and has a different approach to treatment. Urinary incontinence can often be a mixture of more than one type of incontinence. *Stress urinary incontinence* involves accidental leakage of urine with activity, coughing, laughing, and sneezing. This type of incontinence is the most common in men after prostatectomy because they lost part of the mechanisms that maintain urine in the bladder. *Urge incontinence* is an accidental leak of urine associated with a strong urge to urinate. A man with urge incontinence has a sudden, uncontrolled need to urinate. Urge incontinence and urgency can occur after prostate treatment with either radiation or prostatectomy. *Overflow incontinence* occurs when the bladder never empties completely and once it is filled to capacity the urine overflows, causing leakage. This can happen when scar tissue from radiation or surgery obstructs the outlet of the bladder. Some men may also complain of leakage of urine during sexual relations or with orgasm after prostatectomy. Although urine is sterile and a small amount of leakage is not problematic, this problem along with erectile dysfunction after prostate cancer treatment can impair a couple's ability for sex and intimacy.

Treating Incontinence

Incontinence can be treated successfully for the majority of men. Pelvic floor muscle/Kegel exercises are a series of pelvic muscle exercises designed to strengthen the muscles of the pelvic floor. Dr. Arnold Kegel, a gynecologist, developed these exercises in 1948 as a method of controlling incontinence in women after childbirth. Pelvic floor exercises strengthen the muscles of the pelvic floor to improve urethral and rectal sphincter function. The success of pelvic floor exercises depends on proper technique and adhering to a regular exercise program. Pelvic floor muscle exercises can be helpful in treating both urge and stress incontinence. There are both quick and slow-twitch fibers in the pelvic floor muscles and so both quick and slow pelvic floor exercises should be practiced. It is important to do the pelvic floor exercises correctly, and this may require you to see a specialist nurse or physical therapist who can teach you how to do the exercises appropriately and consistently. Your health care provider can also recommend online resources to assist you.

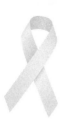

The Agency for Health Care Policy and Research Guideline, *Urinary Incontinence in Adults: Acute and Chronic Management* (Fantl et al., 1996), recommends the primary treatment options for incontinence should be bladder retraining, timed voiding, and pelvic floor exercises. For urge incontinence, there are several prescription anticholinergic medications that may help

The success of pelvic floor exercises depends on proper technique and adhering to a regular exercise program.

control the urge to urinate. There currently are no FDA-approved medications for stress urinary incontinence. Surgical interventions for stress urinary incontinence include various sling procedures and artificial sphincters. Although urinary incontinence is common after prostate cancer treatment, both problems can often (but not always) be treated successfully. It is essential for men with these problems to undergo a full evaluation and treatment of urinary incontinence by a urologic health care provider.

Keys for Success with Pelvic Floor Exercises

✳ The success of pelvic floor exercises depends on proper technique and sticking to a regular exercise program. There are both quick and slow-twitch fibers in the pelvic floor muscles so both quick and slow pelvic floor exercises should be performed.

✳ Do not contract your abdominal, thigh, or buttocks muscles while doing the exercise.

Performing Pelvic Floor Exercises

✳ These suggestions are meant as general guidelines. Ask your provider if he or she has any specific instructions for doing the exercises and how soon after treatment you can do them. Some men may benefit from working with a trained professional such as a nurse or physical therapist who can make sure you are doing the exercises correctly.

✳ Begin by emptying your bladder.

✳ Tighten the pelvic floor muscles and relax them immediately for a quick contraction. Repeat 10 times.

✳ Do 10 slow contractions and relaxations: Holding for 4-5 counts minimum and relaxing for 4-5 counts.

✳ Do three sets a day of both the quick and slow pelvic floor contractions.

✳ Increase contractions by five repetitions each week until you reach a goal of 20-25 quick and 20-25 slow pelvic floor contractions three times a day.

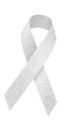

Keys for Success with Pelvic Floor Exercises

(continued)

✳ You can do these exercises at any time and any place. You can do them sitting, standing, or lying down. After 4-6 weeks, most people notice some improvement. It may take as long as 3-4 months to see a major change. Once you feel you are doing much better, drop to one set of 20-25 quick and 20-25 slow contractions a day for maintenance.

✳ *A word of caution:* Some people feel they can speed up the progress by increasing the number of repetitions and the frequency of exercises. However, over-exercising can cause muscle fatigue and increase urine leakage.

✳ When done properly, Kegel exercises may be effective in improving urinary continence.

Notes from discussions with my
provider/caregivers about incontinence.

Chapter 12
The Mind Is the Most Powerful Sex Organ in the Body

You may have heard this phrase before, but it is true. The brain controls everything in our bodies including the various aspects of our sex lives. Men with sexual issues feel a variety of frustrations and concerns about erectile function during sex and this can lead to further erectile issues. Sexual dysfunction after prostate cancer treatment has been associated with decreased health-related quality of life (Hu et al., 2004; Meyer, Gillatt, Lockyer, & Macdonagh, 2003; Penson et al., 2003; Penson et al., 2008; Yarbro & Ferrans, 1998). Sexual dysfunction can impact life satisfaction.

Worrying about erections during sex can lead to further erectile dysfunction.

You may feel many emotions after prostate cancer treatment. After hearing that surgery went well and the cancer was removed, some men feel relief and comfort. Feelings and emotions may vary depending on which treatment you underwent and any side effects such as sexual dysfunction and urinary incontinence. Both urinary incontinence and sexual dysfunction after prostate cancer treatment have been associated with decreased health-related quality of life, depression, and anxiety (Green, Pakenham, Headley, & Gardiner, 2002; Hu et al., 2004; Penson et al., 2008; Wettergren, Bjorkholm, Axdorph, & Langius-Eklof, 2004). Researchers have found that, compared to other treatments, androgen deprivation therapy (hormone ablation therapy) was associated with decreased health-related quality of life and more distress (Couper et al., 2009). It is important to seek help from a qualified professional if you are experiencing ongoing depression and/or anxiety because research has shown treatment can improve your quality of life (Armes et al., 2009; Blank & Bellizzi, 2006; Giesler et al., 2005; Mehnert, Lehmann, Graefen, Huland, & Koch, 2010; Mottet, Prayer-Galetti, Hammerer, Kattan, & Tunn, 2006; Sharpley & Christie, 2009; van den Bergh, Korfage, Borsboom, Steyerberg, & Essink-Bot, 2009).

Intimacy (deeper communication on all levels) is often important to some men and their partners.

Time and Space to Communicate

Worrying about erections during sex can lead to further erectile dysfunction. During sexual stimulation, men need to stay focused on the pleasure of the experience because distractions such as concerns over erectile hardness can be an erection killer. Staying in the moment to enjoy sex is important. Keep the time and space for sexual experiences separate from the time and space when you have discussions about sex. Talking about sexual issues in the heat of the moment during sex will change the focus of your sexual time away from pleasure and arousal.

Some men worry about satisfying a partner and put unneeded importance on the role of erections in bringing sexual pleasure. Talk to your partner about your concerns related to fulfilling her or his needs. Intimacy (deeper communication on all levels) may be more important than sex to some partners.

It is important to talk about sex and to think about where, when, and how you talk about it. Talking about sex may be new and challenging for you and your partner and these discussions take time. Even

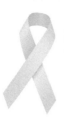

though it is difficult to talk about sex, it will get easier the more you communicate about it. The timing, place, and approach to the sexual discussion can be crucial to successful communication. Plan time for this discussion in a location other than the bedroom or where you are typically sexual. Find a comfortable space away from the bedroom. It may help to sit face-to-face and in close proximity to each other during the discussion. Focus the conversation in terms of your feelings and your needs, using terms such as "I feel frustrated when ___ and I need ___." If you both read this book, discussing the different topics presented will help open up a conversation about sex.

Remember, you are still a vibrant man capable of enjoying sex.

Climax Concerns

Both men and women can climax with or without the man experiencing an erection. Erection is not crucial to sexual satisfaction, and non-penetrative forms of sexual arousal can be very enjoyable for many couples. If you and your partner work together, you can discover new and exciting ways to enjoy your love play together. Focusing on the present moment and pleasure during each of those moments during sex can lead to greater satisfaction, rather than worrying about what is different now. Allow yourself to fully engage in each moment of pleasure during sex and do not let your mind drift to concerns about possible problems. Find a comfortable time to talk to your partner about any worries you may have about problems during sex. These conversations should be ongoing and you both should be comfortable initiating a discussion. Remember, you are still a vibrant man capable of enjoying sex.

Most men do not have problems reaching climax (the good feeling associated with culmination of sex) after prostate treatment. If you have problems climaxing, vibratory stimulation and various nonmedical devices can be effective in helping both men and women reach climax. When a man or woman is struggling with reaching climax, vibratory stimulation is often effective.

One FDA-cleared vibratory medical device, Viberect®, has shown to provoke penile erection and/or ejaculation in spine-injured men and in a very small series of urology patients (10 men total, 5 of which had prostate cancer) with erectile dysfunction. It was found to be safe, easy to use, tolerable, and highly satisfying (Tajkarimi & Burnett, 2012). The device can be costly compared to a nonmedical vibrator, and is available by prescription only. At the time

You are a prostate cancer survivor, and you deserve the best life you can live.

this book was written, there was no published research to support the use of this device so further research is needed.

Seek Support

You may need to grieve the loss resulting from the many changes associated with sex following prostate cancer treatment. Remember, you experienced erections every day of your life since you were born, so a dramatic change in this experience may be upsetting and frustrating. You are entitled to grieve over any loss of function. Other changes such as penile shrinkage, lack of ejaculation, and changes in sensations during climax may also occur and be upsetting. Although most men climax even without erections, sensations may be different for some men and this may be frustrating.

Your feelings are real and valid, and you need to explore those emotions with your partner and other key people in your life. It may also be beneficial to seek professional help from a therapist. Prostate cancer support groups such as Us TOO International can provide needed

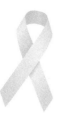
encouragement from other men who have experienced similar challenges. There are Us TOO chapters worldwide. Find one near you and/or consult their online resources. Do not hesitate to seek out whatever resources will help you live a most fulfilling life. You are a prostate cancer survivor, and you deserve the best life you can live.

Chapter 13

A Message for Partners of Men with Erectile Dysfunction after Prostate Cancer Treatment

This chapter is especially for partners of men who have undergone prostate cancer treatment. You have lived through every phase of prostate cancer survival and it has been challenging for both you and your partner. It is not easy to watch someone you love suffer with a prostate cancer diagnosis. Partners often feel like an outside observer experiencing the effects of prostate cancer treatment along with their mate, yet they also feel significant emotional distress themselves. In a study of 1,201 prostate cancer patients treated with surgery or radiation and 625 partners, researchers found that improvement in erectile function may improve health-related quality of life of *both* men with prostate cancer and their partners (Sanda et al., 2008). In a small study from Australia of 50 female partners of men with prostate cancer, women were very resilient in coping with their partner's prostate cancer, but 22% showed signs of depression and anxiety and reduced coping levels (Street et al., 2009).

You may experience a myriad of different feelings at different times. Although prostate cancer is very survivable, there can be many difficulties in dealing with side effects of treatment. It is not unusual to feel insecure about affection, intimacy, and sex. Sometimes you can become so concerned about upsetting your partner that you stop being physical and affectionate. Both of you need to find a way to be physically and emotionally supportive of each other. If you and your

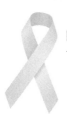

partner do not talk about these feelings and vulnerabilities, you will not understand your partner's needs in terms of support. Your partner can not understand your vulnerabilities and needs if you do not communicate those issues to him. Support in terms of emotional and physical affection is very important to both you and your partner.

Communicate

It is important to discuss your feelings and communicate concerns about physical contact. This may be something new for both you and your partner since many people do not talk about sex very much. Communication can be key to decreasing misunderstanding. Your loving and accepting approach to your partner can decrease the pressure he puts on himself about sexual performance. Let you partner know that affection and intimacy are important too and are not compromised by erectile dysfunction. You and your partner can cuddle and be sexual in ways that do not require erections. All sex can be enjoyable and most men and their partners can climax without penetrative sex. Climax is independent of erections and men who have erectile dysfunction from prostate cancer treatment are typically able to climax pleasurably without difficulty.

It is important to discuss your feelings and communicate concerns about physical contact.

Think of this experience as a fresh opportunity to discover new ways to be sexual and bring pleasure to each other. Erections are not needed for oral or manual sexual stimulation and many techniques can be enjoyable for you and your partner. With the attitude that "it is all enjoyable," you and your partner can enjoy sexual exploration and affection in new ways. If erections happen, that is great; but if erections do not happen, sex can still be very enjoyable. Remember, an erection is not essential to sexual enjoyment.

Maintaining Attraction

As discussed earlier, the goal of penile rehabilitation is to improve blood flow to the penis while the nerves recover after prostate surgery or during diminished erectile function after radiation therapy. Men who have undergone prostate cancer treatment are using erectile treatments to improve penile blood flow and preserve erectile function. Regular use of medications or the vacuum device may improve penile blood flow. You can help your partner by encouraging him to use these treatments along with regular stimulation to promote penile blood flow. Your partner may be embarrassed about needing to regularly self-stimulate and may desire some help from you.

You also have sexual needs and concerns, and it may be important for you to think about how you can deal with your own sexual desires while being supportive to your partner. Many men with erectile dysfunction worry about meeting their partner's needs. Communication about these topics can alleviate some fears and concerns. Attraction towards each other does not have to be impacted by prostate cancer. Letting each other know that you remain attracted to each other and that you find each other sexy can improve sexual self-esteem. It is important to continue to be affectionate and have fun in the many ways you always had fun together. Your attraction to each other and sexual life together are unique characteristics that set your relationship apart from your relationship with others, so maintaining these aspects of your relationship is very important.

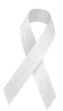

Seek Help

Partners may also find that they have their own sexual issues. It is not unusual for women to have changes in desire and arousal before, during, and after menopause. Common problems include vaginal dryness, stress urinary incontinence, changes in ability to become stimulated, and difficulty reaching climax. Diminishing hormones such as estrogen and testosterone can cause some of these problems. Many men experience erectile dysfunction related to medical conditions that occur in the later years of life, such as diabetes, high cholesterol, high blood pressure, heart disease, and obesity. Some men also experience diminished sexual desire. It is important for you (just like your partner with prostate cancer) to speak to a health care professional about these problems as many of them can be addressed successfully.

Partners may also find that they have their own sexual issues.

Chapter 14

Dealing with Challenges Related to Decreased Mobility or Losing Erections in Different Positions

Although sex does not take much more exertion than the energy to climb stairs or carry a heavy bag of groceries, it does take effort and you do burn calories. As a general rule, if you can safely climb two flights of 5-10 steps comfortably without chest pain, you can probably engage in intercourse (but if you have a heart condition or other medical conditions, consult your doctor before engaging in sexual activities). Some positions and activities may become more challenging as your mobility decreases or you experience other physical limitations. You might try an intercourse position that requires less energy such as lying

Sex can be very fulfilling after prostate cancer treatment, even though it may be different.

side by side or sitting with your partner in your lap. If one partner has more energy or stamina than the other, that partner may be better able to handle the capacity requirements of being on top during intercourse. These positions may be better for couples with decreased energy levels or conditions that affect stamina.

You also may experience better erections in upright positions. Although you may prefer certain positions (those you have used your entire life during sex), others may work better in cases of erectile dysfunction. If you are on top of your partner, your penis gets more blood and may remain harder. The penis may also be harder when

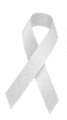
you are standing or kneeling rather than lying down. Your partner may kneel and you can have intercourse from behind in a more upright position. Using a tension ring device during sex may help maintain an erect penis in various positions.

Trying different positions or ways of being sexual can be exciting and fun.

Sex can be very fulfilling after prostate cancer treatment, even though it may be different. Trying different positions or ways of being sexual can be exciting and fun, or you can allow yourself to become frustrated and upset that things are different now. If your erections are not being cooperative, you can still be sexual with your partner. Oral or manual sexual stimulation can be very enjoyable and lead to climax. The keys to enjoying sex in different ways are open communication with your partner, willingness to explore and enjoy each other in different ways, and working together to try positions or sexual stimulation that is enjoyable for both of you.

Chapter 15
Conclusion: Be Informed

Erectile dysfunction is one of the most common adverse side effects following prostate cancer treatment. Although some men might not be concerned about erectile function, others are distressed about this problem and need assistance in determining the best way to move forward to promote and preserve erectile health. Each treatment option has both positive and negative aspects. Ultimately, you must make the best-informed decision for yourself. You need to decide how and if you want to treat erectile dysfunction, and make choices regarding penile rehabilitation and promoting blood flow to your penis to encourage return of spontaneous erections. Each man has his own unique sexual expression. Together you and your health care professional can carefully determine how a potential treatment would work within your life.

Together you and your health care professional can carefully determine how a potential treatment would work within your life.

Penile rehabilitation may improve return of spontaneous erections and your response to some ED treatments. However, there is no clear evidence to support any particular treatment for ED or penile rehabilitation. So, you must look at the pros and cons of each treatment and make decisions that are best for you and your partner. Generally, patients tend to start with less-invasive or less-cumbersome options. Most men prefer oral agents because they are discreet and easy to utilize, and these medications can be a first-line treatment. Keep in mind that failure rates for oral agents are very high in men after

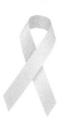

prostate removal and sometimes after radiation therapy. You will probably need more effective options instead of the oral agents (or in combination with them) to provide sufficient erectile function for sex. Nevertheless, despite the fact that oral agents do not always provide sufficient erectile rigidity for penetrative sex, they may provide improved return of spontaneous erections after prostate cancer treatments (Montorsi et al., 2000; Schwartz, Wong, & Graydon, 2004). In addition, other treatments such as the vacuum device or MUSE can be used in conjunction with the oral agents to enhance erections and penile rehabilitation.

As a next step, some patients may prefer a less-invasive treatment such as the vacuum constriction device. Although the vacuum device is the least-invasive treatment option, it is cumbersome, requires the user to wear a tension ring during sex, and entails much patience and work to master the use of the device. Another less-invasive treatment that is simple to use is MUSE. An important factor about MUSE to keep in mind is the issue of pain with alprostadil use after radical prostatectomy.

If you are looking for efficacy and are motivated to carefully use a treatment that is a little more invasive, injections may be an option. You need to understand serious complications are rare, but may occur with this therapy. If you are motivated to regularly prepare and give yourself the injection, this treatment provides consistently effective erections that feel and look fairly close to natural erections. Finally, when medical treatments have failed, it is time to consider the penile implant. The implant provides an effective treatment that is associated with high patient and partner satisfaction, but not all men are willing to undergo this surgical intervention.

Importance of Treatment

It is critically important you understand that *not* utilizing any treatment to promote cavernosal blood flow and oxygenation may have long-term ramifications for regaining erectile function in the future. Each year research continues to reveal the importance of using treatment for erectile dysfunction to promote corporal tissue health and diminish atrophic changes to the penile tissue. After prostate surgery, nitric oxide synthesis is diminished due to nerve trauma to the cavernosal nerve (Carrier et al., 1995). The lack of nitric oxide and neuropraxia (nerve no longer transmits impulses) lead to diminished blood flow and oxygenation of the penile tissue, which leads to cavernosal fibrosis and collagen synthesis (Leungwattanakij et al., 2003). Atrophy and penile fibrosis cause further erectile dysfunction after radical prostatectomy. Therefore, re-establishing blood flow to the penis is important to preserve and promote optimal erectile function following prostate cancer treatment. The advent of earlier rehabilitation supports better return of spontaneous erectile function, or at least erectile dysfunction that can be treated with less-invasive therapies such as the oral medications.

Sex and intimacy need not be lost following treatment of your prostate cancer.

By understanding each treatment option and determining the best choice for treatment, you can find the optimal treatment option for erectile dysfunction and penile rehabilitation. As you consider options, carefully consider your unique sexual lifestyle and how you will incorporate erectile dysfunction treatment into your sexual experience. This important component of life need not be lost following treatment of your prostate cancer.

References

Albaugh, J.A. (2006). Intracavernosal injection algorithm. *Urologic Nursing, 26*(6), 449-453.

Albaugh, J.A., & Ferrans, C.E. (2009). Patient reported pain associated with initial intracavernosal injection. *Journal of Sexual Medicine, 6*(2), 513-519.

Albaugh, J.A., & Ferrans, C.E. (2010). Impact of penile injections on patients with erectile dysfunction after prostatectomy. *Urologic Nursing, 30*(3), 167-178.

Armes, J., Crowe, M., Colbourne, L., Morgan, H., Murrells, T., Oakley, C., ... Richardson, A. (2009). Patients' supportive care needs beyond the end of cancer treatment: a prospective, longitudinal survey. *Journal of Clinical Oncology, 27*(36), 6172-6179.

Baniel, J., Israilov, S., Engelstein, D., Shmueli, J., Segenreich, E., & Livne, P.M. (2000). Three-year outcome of a progressive treatment program for erectile dysfunction with intracavernous injections of vasoactive drugs. *Urology, 56*(4), 647-652.

Baniel, J., Israilov, S., Segenreich, E., & Livne, P. M. (2001). Comparative evaluation of treatments for erectile dysfunction in patients with prostate cancer after radical retropubic prostatectomy. *British Journal of Urology International, 88*(1), 58-62.

Bannowsky, A., Schulze, H., van der Horst, C., Hautmann, S., & Junemann, K.P. (2008). Recovery of erectile function after nerve-sparing radical prostatectomy: Improvement with nightly low-dose sildenafil. *British Journal of Urology International, 101*(10), 1279-1283.

Bennett, A.H., Carpenter, A.J., & Barada, J.H. (1991). An improved vasoactive drug combination for a pharmacological erection program. *Journal of Urology, 146*(6), 1564-1565.

Blank, T.O., & Bellizzi, K.M. (2006). After prostate cancer: Predictors of well-being among long-term prostate cancer survivors. *Cancer, 106*(10), 2128-2135.

Carrier, S., Zvara, P., Nunes, L., Kour, N.W., Rehman, J., & Lue, T.F. (1995). Regeneration of nitric oxide synthase-containing nerves after cavernous nerve neurotomy in the rat. *Journal of Urology, 153*(5), 1722-1727.

Chen, J., Sofer, M., Kaver, I., Matzkin, H., & Greenstein, A. (2004). Concomitant use of sildenafil and a vacuum entrapment device for the treatment of erectile dysfunction. *Journal of Urology, 171*(1), 292-295.

Claro Jde, A., de Aboim, J. E., Maringolo, M., Andrade, E., Aguiar, W., Nogueira, M., ... Srougi, M. (2001). Intracavernous injection in the treatment of erectile dysfunction after radical prostatectomy: An observational study. *Sao Paulo Medical Journal, 119*(4), 135-137.

Cookson, M.S., & Nadig, P.W. (1993). Long-term results with vacuum constriction device. *Journal of Urology, 149*(2), 290-294.

Costabile, R.A., Spevak, M., Fishman, I.J., Govier, F.E., Hellstrom, W.J., Shabsigh, R., … Gesundheit, N. (1998). Efficacy and safety of transurethral alprostadil in patients with erectile dysfunction following radical prostatectomy. *Journal of Urology, 160*(4), 1325-1328.

Couper, J.W., Love, A.W., Dunai, J.V., Duchesne, G.M., Bloch, S., Costello, A.J., & Kissane, D.W. (2009). The psychological aftermath of prostate cancer treatment choices: A comparison of depression, anxiety and quality of life outcomes over the 12 months following diagnosis. *Medical Journal of Australia, 190*(7 Suppl.), S86-89.

Dennis, R.L., & McDougal, W.S. (1988). Pharmacological treatment of erectile dysfunction after radical prostatectomy. *Journal of Urology, 139*(4), 775-776.

El-Hakim, A., & Tweari, A. (2004). Robotic prostatectomy - a review. *Medscape General Medicine, 6*(4), 20.

Fantl, J.A. and the Urinary Incontinence in Adults Guideline Panel. (1996). *Urinary incontinence in adults: Acute and chronic management.* AHCPR Publication No. 96-0682. Rockville, MD: U.S. Department of Health and Human Services.

Frankel, S.J., Donovan, J.L., Peters, T.I., Abrams, P., Dabhoiwala, N.F., Osawa, D., & Lin, A.T. (1998). Sexual dysfunction in men with lower urinary tract symptoms. *Journal of Clinical Epidemiology, 51*(8), 677-685.

Gerstenberg, T.C., Metz, P., Ottesen, B., & Fahrenkrug, J. (1992). Intracavernous self-injection with vasoactive intestinal polypeptide and phentolamine in the management of erectile failure. *Journal of Urology, 147*(5), 1277-1279.

Giesler, R.B., Given, B., Given, C.W., Rawl, S., Monahan, P., Burns, D., … Champion, V. (2005). Improving the quality of life of patients with prostate carcinoma: A randomized trial testing the efficacy of a nurse-driven intervention. *Cancer, 104*(4), 752-762.

Gontero, P., Fontana, F., Bagnasacco, A., Panella, M., Kocjancic, E., Pretti, G., & Frea, B. (2003). Is there an optimal time for intracavernous prostaglandin E1 rehabilitation following nonnerve sparing radical prostatectomy? Results from a hemodynamic prospective study. *Journal of Urology, 169*(6), 2166-2169.

Gould, J.E., Switters, D.M., Broberick, G.A., & deVereWhite, R.W. (1992). External vacuum devices: A clinical comparison with pharmacologic erections. *World Journal of Urology, 10,* 68-70.

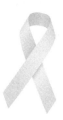

Green, H.J., Pakenham, K.I., Headley, B.C., & Gardiner, R.A. (2002). Coping and health-related quality of life in men with prostate cancer randomly assigned to hormonal medication or close monitoring. *Psychooncology, 11*(5), 401-414.

Hatfield, E. (1982). Passionate love, companionate love, and intimacy. In M. Fisher & G. Stricker (Eds.), *Intimacy* (pp. 267-292). New York, NY: Plenum.

Hatzimouratidis, K., Burnett, A.L., Hatzichristou, D., McCullough, A.R., Montorsi, F., & Mulhall, J.P. (2009). Phosphodiesterase type 5 inhibitors in postprostatectomy erectile dysfunction: A critical analysis of the basic science rationale and clinical application. *European Urology, 55*(2), 334-347.

Hu, J.C., Elkin, E.P., Pasta, D.J., Lubeck, D.P., Kattan, M.W., Carroll, P.R., & Litwin, M.S. (2004). Predicting quality of life after radical prostatectomy: Results from CaPSURE. *Journal of Urology, 171*(2 Pt 1), 703-707; discussion 707-708.

Incrocci, L., Koper, P.C., Hop, W.C., & Slob, A.K. (2001). Sildenafil citrate (Viagra) and erectile dysfunction following external beam radiotherapy for prostate cancer: A randomized, double-blind, placebo-controlled, cross-over study. *International Journal of Radiation Oncology, Biology, and Physics, 51*(5), 1190-1195.

Incrocci, L., Slagter, C., Slob, A.K., & Hop, W.C. (2006). A randomized, double-blind, placebo-controlled, cross-over study to assess the efficacy of tadalafil (Cialis) in the treatment of erectile dysfunction following three-dimensional conformal external-beam radiotherapy for prostatic carcinoma. *International Journal of Radiation Oncology, Biology, and Physics, 66*(2), 439-444.

Jacobsen, N.E., Moore, K.N., Estey, E., & Voaklander, D. (2007). Open versus laparoscopic radical prostatectomy: A prospective comparison of postoperative urinary incontinence rates. *Journal of Urology, 177*(2), 615-619.

Jardin, A., Wagner, G., Khoury, S., Giuliano, F., Padma-Nathan, H., & Rosen, R. (2000). *Erectile dysfunction: 1st international consultation on erectile dysfunction.* Plymouth, United Kingdom: Plymbridge Distributors Ltd.

Kohler, T.S., Pedro, R., Hendlin, K., Utz, W., Ugarte, R., Reddy, P., ... Monga, M. (2007). A pilot study on the early use of the vacuum erection device after radical retropubic prostatectomy. *British Journal of Urology International, 100*(4), 858-862.

Korfage, I.J., Essink-Bot, M.L., Borsboom, G.J., Madalinska, J.B., Kirkels, W.J., Habbema, J.D., ... de Koning, H.J. (2005). Five-year follow-up of health-related quality of life after primary treatment of localized prostate cancer. *International Journal of Cancer. Journal International du Cancer, 116*(2), 291-296.

Leungwattanakij, S., Bivalacqua, T.J., Usta, M.F., Yang, D.Y., Hyun, J.S., Champion, H.C., ... Hellstrom, W.J. (2003). Cavernous neurotomy causes hypoxia and fibrosis in rat corpus cavernosum. *Journal of Andrology, 24*(2), 239-245.

McCullough, A.R. (2007). The effect of low dose intraurethral alprostadil (MUSE®) on corporal oxygenation after nerve sparing radical prostatectomy: 77. *Journal of Sexual Medicine, 4*(1 Suppl.), 89.

McCullough, A.R., Levine, L.A., & Padma-Nathan, H. (2008). Return of nocturnal erections and erectile function after bilateral nerve-sparing radical prostatectomy in men treated nightly with sildenafil citrate: Subanalysis of a longitudinal randomized double-blind placebo-controlled trial. *Journal of Sexual Medicine, 5*(2), 476-484.

McMahon, C.G., Samali, R., & Johnson, H. (2000). Efficacy, safety and patient acceptance of sildenafil citrate as treatment for erectile dysfunction. *The Journal of Urology, 164*(4), 1192-1196.

Mehnert, A., Lehmann, C., Graefen, M., Huland, H., & Koch, U. (2010). Depression, anxiety, post-traumatic stress disorder and health-related quality of life and its association with social support in ambulatory prostate cancer patients. *European Journal of Cancer Care (England), 19*(6), 736-745.

Menon, M., Kaul, S., Bhandari, A., Shrivastava, A., Tewari, A., & Hemal, A. (2005). Potency following robotic radical prostatectomy: A questionnaire based analysis of outcomes after conventional nerve sparing and prostatic fascia sparing techniques. *The Journal of Urology, 174*(6), 2291-2296.

Menon, M., Shrivastava, A., Kaul, S., Badani, K. K., Fumo, M., Bhandari, M., & Peabody, J.O. (2007). Vattikuti Institute prostatectomy: Contemporary technique and analysis of results. *European Urology, 51*(3), 648-657; discussion 657-648.

Meyer, J.P., Gillatt, D.A., Lockyer, R., & Macdonagh, R. (2003). The effect of erectile dysfunction on the quality of life of men after radical prostatectomy. *British Journal of Urology International, 92*(9), 929-931.

Miller, D.C., Wei, J.T., Dunn, R.L., Montie, J.E., Pimentel, H., Sandler, H.M., ... Sanda, M.G. (2006). Use of medications or devices for erectile dysfunction among long-term prostate cancer treatment survivors: Potential influence of sexual motivation and/or indifference. *Urology, 68*(1), 166-171.

Montague, D.K., & Angermeier, K.W. (2000). Current status of penile prosthesis implantation. *Current Urology Reports, 1*(4), 291-296.

Montague, D.K., & Angermeier, K.W. (2003). Contemporary aspects of penile prosthesis implantation. *Urologia Internationalis, 70*(2), 141-146.

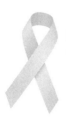

Montorsi, F., Brock, G., Lee, J., Shapiro, J., Van Poppel, H., Graefen, M., & Stief, C. (2008). Effect of nightly versus on-demand vardenafil on recovery of erectile function in men following bilateral nerve-sparing radical prostatectomy. *European Urology, 54*(4), 924-931.

Montorsi, F., Guazzoni, G., Strambi, L. F., Da Pozzo, L. F., Nava, L., Barbieri, L., ... Mlani, A. (1997). Recovery of spontaneous erectile function after nerve-sparing radical retropubic prostatectomy with and without early intracavernous injections of alprostadil: Results of a prospective, randomized trial. [see comment]. *Journal of Urology, 158*(4), 1408-1410.

Montorsi, F., Maga, T., Strambi, L. F., Salonia, A., Barbieri, L., Scattoni, V., ... Pizzini, G. (2000). Sildenafil taken at bedtime significantly increases nocturnal erections: results of a placebo-controlled study. *Urology, 56*(6), 906-911.

Montorsi, F., Salonia, A., Zanoni, M., Pompa, P., Cestari, A., Guazzoni, G., ... Rigatti, P. (2002). Current status of local penile therapy. *International Journal of Impotence Research, 14*(Suppl. 1), S70-81.

Mottet, N., Prayer-Galetti, T., Hammerer, P., Kattan, M.W., & Tunn, U. (2006). Optimizing outcomes and quality of life in the hormonal treatment of prostate cancer. *BJU International, 98*(1), 20-27.

Mulhall, J.P. (2008). Penile rehabilitation following radical prostatectomy. *Current Opinion in Urology, 18*(6), 613-620.

Mulhall, J.P., Jahoda, A.E., Cairney, M., Goldstein, B., Leitzes, R., Woods, J., ... Goldstein, I. (1999). The causes of patient dropout from penile self-injection therapy for impotence. *Journal of Urology, 162*(4), 1291-1294.

Mulhall, J.P., Land, S., Parker, M., Waters, W.B., & Flanigan, R.C. (2005). The use of an erectogenic pharmacotherapy regimen following radical prostatectomy improves recovery of spontaneous erectile function. *Journal of Sexual Medicine, 2*(4), 532-540; discussion 540-532.

Mulligan, T., & Moss, C.R. (1991). Sexuality and aging in male veterans: A cross sectional study of interest, ability, and activity. *Archives of Sexual Behavior, 20,* 17-25.

Nandipati, K.C., Raina, R., Agarwal, A., & Zippe, C.D. (2006). Erectile dysfunction following radical retropubic prostatectomy: Epidemiology, pathophysiology and pharmacological management. *Drugs and Aging, 23*(2), 101-117.

NIH Consensus Development Panel on Impotence. (1993). NIH consensus conference. Impotence. NIH consensus development panel on impotence. *Journal of the American Medical Association, 270*(1), 83-90.

Nehra, A., Blute, M.L., Barrett, D.M., & Moreland, R.B. (2002). Rationale for combination therapy of intraurethral prostaglandin E(1) and sildenafil in the salvage of erectile dysfunction patients desiring noninvasive therapy. *International Journal of Impotence Research, 14*(Suppl. 1), S38-S42.

Padma-Nathan, H., McCullough, A.R., Giuliano, F., Toler, S.M., Wohlhuter, C., & Shplisky, A.B. (2003). Postoperative nightly administration of sildenafil citrate significantly improved the return of normal spontaneous erectile function after bilateral nerve-sparing radical retropubic prostatectomy with and without early intracavernous injections of alprostadil: Results of a prospective, randomized trial. *Journal of Urology, 169*(4 Suppl.), 375-376.

Padmanaban, P., & McCullough, A. (2006). The effect of prostaglandin E-1 (PGE-1) urethral suppository (MUSE) and injections on corporal oxygenation saturation (stO2) in men with erectile dysfunction. *Journal of Andrology, 27*(Abstract).

Penson, D.F., Latini, D.M., Lubeck, D.P., Wallace, K., Henning, J.M., & Lue, T. (2003). Is quality of life different for men with erectile dysfunction and prostate cancer compared to men with erectile dysfunction due to other causes? Results from the ExCEED data base. *Journal of Urology, 169*(4), 1458-1461.

Penson, D.F., McLerran, D., Feng, Z., Li, L., Albertsen, P.C., Gilliland, F.D., … Stanford, J.L. (2005). 5-year urinary and sexual outcomes after radical prostatectomy: Results from the prostate cancer outcomes study. *The Journal of Urology, 173*(5), 1701-1705.

Penson, D.F., McLerran, D., Feng, Z., Li, L., Albertsen, P.C., Gilliland, F.D., … Standford, J.L. (2008). 5-year urinary and sexual outcomes after radical prostatectomy: Results from the Prostate Cancer Outcomes Study. *Journal of Urology, 179*(5 Suppl.), S40-44.

Porst, H. (1996). The rationale for prostaglandin E1 in erectile failure: A survey of worldwide experience. *Journal of Urology, 155*(3), 802-815.

Porst, H., Buvat, J., Meuleman, E., Michal, V., & Wagner, G. (1998). Intracavernous alprostadil Alfadex – an effective and well tolerated treatment for erectile dysfunction. Results of a long-term European study. *International Journal of Impotence Research, 10*(4), 225-231.

Potosky, A.L., Davis, W.W., Hoffman, R.M., Stanford, J.L., Stephenson, R.A., Penson, D.F., & Harlan, L.C. (2004). Five-year outcomes after prostatectomy or radiotherapy for prostate cancer: The prostate cancer outcomes study. *Journal of the National Cancer Institute, 96*(18), 1358-1367.

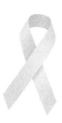

Purvis, K., Egdetveit, I., & Christiansen, E. (1999). Intracavernosal therapy for erectile failure – impact of treatment and reasons for drop-out and dissatisfaction. *International Journal of Impotence Research, 11*(5), 287-299.

Raina, R., Agarwal, A., Allamaneni, S.S., Lakin, M.M., & Zippe, C.D. (2005). Sildenafil citrate and vacuum constriction device combination enhances sexual satisfaction in erectile dysfunction after radical prostatectomy. *Urology, 65*(2), 360-364.

Raina, R., Agarwal, A., Ausmundson, S., Lakin, M., Nandipati, K.C., Montague, D.K., ... Zippe, C.D. (2006). Early use of vacuum constriction device following radical prostatectomy facilitates early sexual activity and potentially earlier return of erectile function. *International Journal of Impotence Research, 18*(1), 77-81.

Raina, R., Agarwal, A., Nandipati, K., & Zippe, C. (2005). Interim analysis of the early use of MUSE following radical prostatectomy (RP) to facilitate early sexual activity and return of spontaneous erectile function. *Journal of Urology, 173*(Suppl.), Abstract 737.

Raina, R., Agarwal, A., Zaramo, C.E., Ausmundson, S., Mansour, D., & Zippe, C.D. (2005). Long-term efficacy and compliance of MUSE for erectile dysfunction following radical prostatectomy: SHIM (IIEF-5) analysis. *International Journal of Impotence Research, 17*(1), 86-90.

Raina, R., Lakin, M.M., Thukral, M., Agarwal, A., Ausmundson, S., Montague, D.K., ... Zippe, C.D. (2003). Long-term efficacy and compliance of intracorporeal (IC) injection for erectile dysfunction following radical prostatectomy: SHIM (IIEF-5) analysis. *International Journal of Impotence Research, 15*(5), 318-322.

Raina, R., Nandipati, K.C., Agarwal, A., Mansour, D., Kaelber, D.C., & Zippe, C.D. (2005). Combination therapy: Medicated urethral system for erection enhances sexual satisfaction in sildenafil citrate failure following nerve-sparing radical prostatectomy. *Journal of Andrology, 26*(6), 757-760.

Raina, R., Pahlajani, G., Agarwal, A., & Zippe, C. D. (2008). Early penile rehabilitation following radical prostatectomy: Cleveland Clinic experience. *International Journal of Impotence Research, 20*(2), 121-126.

Ramsawh, H.J., Morgentaler, A., Covino, N., Barlow, D.H., & DeWolf, W.C. (2005). Quality of life following simultaneous placement of penile prosthesis with radical prostatectomy. *Journal of Urology, 174*(4 Pt 1), 1395-1398.

Sacco, E., Prayer-Galetti, T., Pinto, F., Fracalanza, S., Betto, G., Pagano, F., & Artibani, W. (2006). Urinary incontinence after radical prostatectomy: Incidence by definition, risk factors and temporal trend in a large series with a long-term follow-up. *British Journal of Urology International, 97*(6), 1234-1241.

Sanda, M.G., Dunn, R.L., Michalski, J., Sandler, H.M., Northouse, L., Hembroff, L., … Wei, J.T. (2008). Quality of life and satisfaction with outcome among prostate-cancer survivors. *New England Journal of Medicine, 358*(12), 1250-1261.

Sandhu, D., Curless, E., Dean, J., Hackett, G., Liu, S., Savage, D., … Frentz, G. (1999). A double blind, placebo controlled study of intracavernosal vasoactive intestinal polypeptide and phenotolamine mesylate in a novel auto-injector for the treatment of non-psychogenic erectile dysfunction. *International Journal of Impotence Research, 11*(2), 91-97.

Schwartz, E.J., Wong, P., & Graydon, R.J. (2004). Sildenafil preserves intracorporeal smooth muscle after radical retropubic prostatectomy. *Journal of Urology, 171*(2 Pt 1), 771-774.

Schwarz Pharma. (2004). *Edex (alprostadil) prescribing information.* Milwaukee, WI: Schwarz Pharma.

Seyam, R., Mohamed, K., Al Akhras, A., & Rashwan, H. (2005). A prospective randomized study to optimize the dosage of trimix ingredients and compare its efficacy and safety with prostaglandin E1. *International Journal of Impotence Research, 17,* 346-353.

Shah, P.J., Dinsmore, W., Oakes, R.A., & Hackett, G. (2007). Injection therapy for the treatment of erectile dysfunction: A comparison between alprostadil and a combination of vasoactive intestinal polypeptide and phentolamine mesilate. *Current Medical Research and Opinion, 23*(10), 2577-2583.

Sharpley, C.F., & Christie, D.R. (2009). Effects of interval between diagnosis and time of survey upon preferred information format for prostate cancer patients. *Journal of Medical Imaging and Radiation Oncology, 53*(2), 221-225.

Soderdahl, D.W., Thrasher, J.B., & Hansberry, K.L. (1997). Intracavernosal drug-induced erection therapy versus external vacuum devices in the treatment of erectile dysfunction. *British Journal of Urology, 79*(6), 952-957.

Street, A.F., Couper, J.W., Love, A.W., Bloch, S., Kissane, D.W., & Street, B.C. (2009). Psychosocial adaptation in female partners of men with prostate cancer. *European Journal of Cancer Care, 19*(2), 234-242.

Tajkarimi, K., & Burnett, A.L. (2012). Viberect device use by men with erectile dysfunction: Safety, ease of use, tolerability and satisfaction survey. *Journal of Sexual Medicine, 9*(Suppl. 1), 55.

Tal, R., Teloken, P., & Mulhall, J. P. (2011). Erectile function rehabilitation after radical prostatectomy: Practice patterns among AUA members. *Journal of Sexual Medicine, 8*(8), 2370-2376.

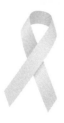

Turner, L.A., Althof, S.E., Levine, S.B., Bodner, D.R., Kursh, E.D., & Resnick, M.I. (1991). External vacuum devices in the treatment of erectile dysfunction: A one-year study of sexual and psychosocial impact. *Journal of Sex and Marital Therapy, 17*(2), 81-93.

Turner, L.A., Althof, S.E., Levine, S.B., Bodner, D.R., Kursh, E.D., & Resnick, M.I. (1992). Twelve-month comparison of two treatments for erectile dysfunction: Self-injection versus external vacuum devices. *Urology, 39*(2), 139-144.

van den Bergh, R.C., Korfage, I.J., Borsboom, G.J., Steyerberg, E.W., & Essink-Bot, M.L. (2009). Prostate cancer-specific anxiety in Dutch patients on active surveillance: Validation of the Memorial Anxiety Scale for Prostate Cancer. *Quality of Life Research, 18*(8), 1061-1066.

Walsh, P.C., Marschke, P., Ricker, D., & Burnett, A.L. (2000). Patient-reported urinary continence and sexual function after anatomic radical prostatectomy. *Urology, 55*(1), 58-61.

Walsh, P.C., & Mostwin, J.L. (1984). Radical prostatectomy and cystoprostatectomy with preservation of potency. Results using a new nerve-sparing technique. *British Journal of Urology, 56*(6), 694-697.

Wettergren, L., Bjorkholm, M., Axdorph, U., & Langius-Eklof, A. (2004). Determinants of health-related quality of life in long-term survivors of Hodgkin's lymphoma. *Quality of Life Research, 13*(8), 1369-1379.

Witherington, R. (1989). Vacuum constriction device for management of erectile impotence. *Journal of Urology, 141*(2), 320-322.

Yarbro, C.H., & Ferrans, C.E. (1998). Quality of life of patients with prostate cancer treated with surgery or radiation therapy. *Oncology Nursing Forum, 25*(4), 685-693.

Zippe, C.D., Raina, R., Thukral, M., Lakin, M.M., Klein, E.A., & Agarwal, A. (2001). Management of erectile dysfunction following radical prostatectomy. *Current Urology Reports, 2*(6), 495-503.